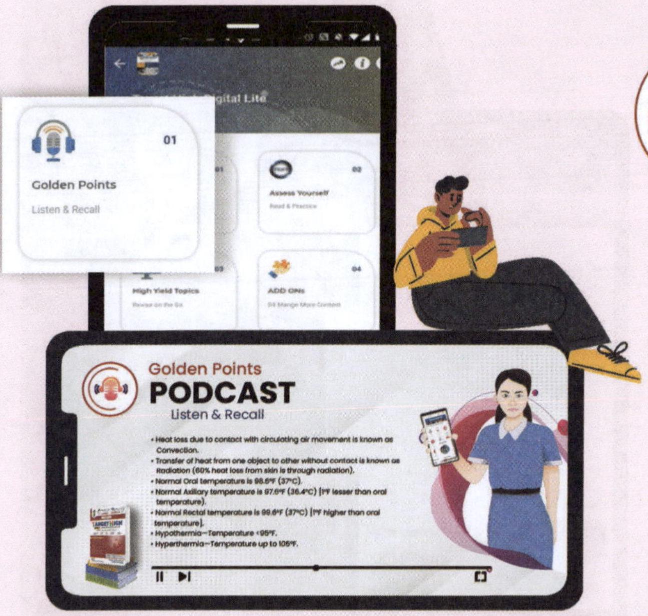

Golden Points Podcast

Listen & Recall

Get

3000+

Golden Points in Podcast Form

(Covering important one-liners from all the subjects)

Elevate Your Learning Skills Through Active Listening

With **AMLI** (*The* **TH** *Educator*)

DON'T FORGET TO

Assess Yourself

Read & Practice

Success Rises With Every Question: Practice for Achievement

Get Yourself Assessed with

AMLI

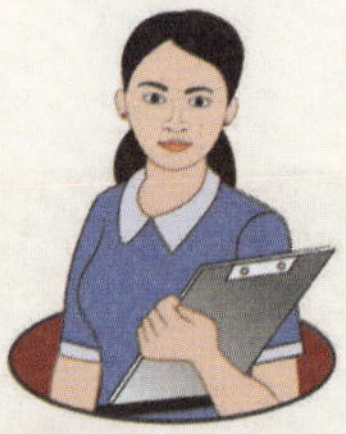

80+ Tests

(Subject-wise Tests & IBQ tests)

covering **8000+ Questions**

48 Grand Tests

based on **new exam pattern of NORCET (Pre/Mains)**

covering **4800 questions**

Real-time Approach and National Level Ranking

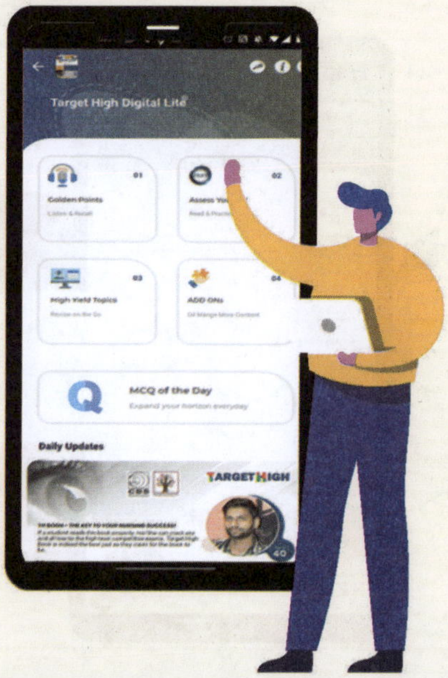

Make your prep easy with Target High Hybrid Digital Edition
The content in this book is excellent, comprehensive and informative. It contains quality MCQs with rationales that will push the registered nurses toward their Targets. Now it is in Hybrid form - Target High Digital Lite which makes your nursing competitive exams prep easy.
Sunil Kumar Choudhary *(Nagaur, Rajasthan)*

A concoction of Nursing excellence!
The Target High Hybrid book is a unique compendium covering all the important subjects needed to excel in your staff nurse entrance exams. The content is well explained. There are ample IBQs and previous year papers in the application and book that will make your learning journey highly efficient.
Rakesh Kumar Yadav *(Behror, Rajasthan)*

Download the App
Nursing Next Live

Access
TARGET HIGH Digital Lite

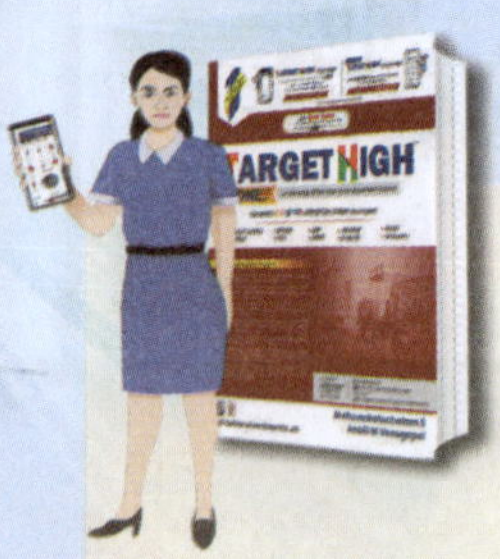

High Yield Topics

Revise on the Go...

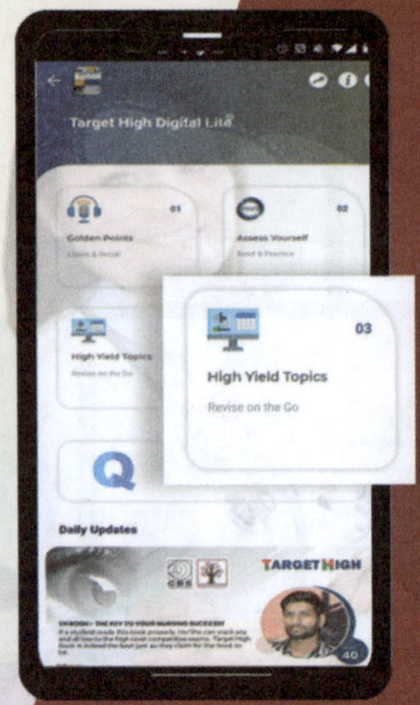

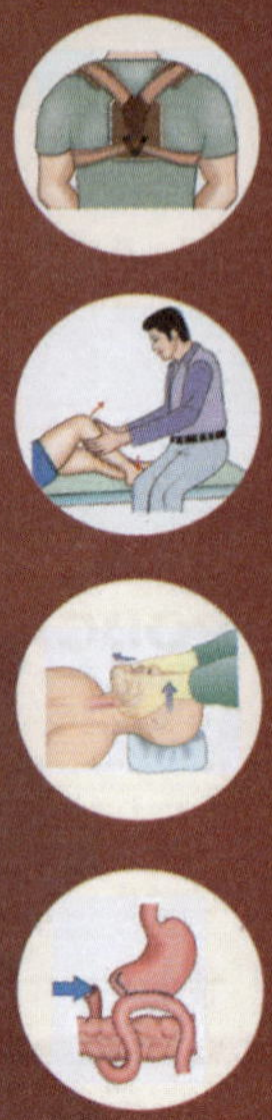

Get Important

300+

High-Yield Topics

(Subject-wise important Tables and Images) with their descriptions for quick access at your Fingertips

Get

Add ONs

Dil Mange More Content

Unleash Your Potential For Free: Dive Into Extra Learning Content

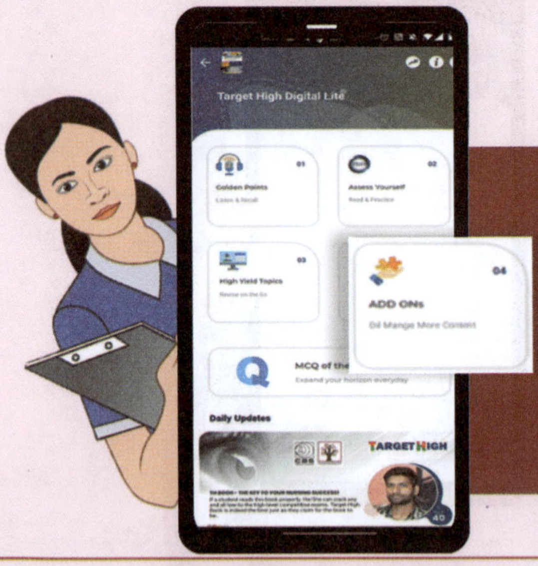

- **115+** Previous Year Papers (from 2023-2004) of all State/ National Level Exam) including NORCET. Selective Papers are given with Rationale.
- **75+** Appendices
- **Study Plan** – Decoding the case scenario-based questions?
- How to prepare for NORCET – Pre & Mains (an overview)
- Monthly Current Affairs
- Nursing Skill Procedures
- How to Crack Nursing Competitive Exams & Interview Section

THE BEST IS HERE!
The Hybrid feature of Target High is more than enough: It has any doubt, ask AMLI feature, ""be in Spotlight"" that highlights the rank holders, current affairs in dil mange more, and many more to make your learning journey highly effective.

Shankar Raj (*Nalanda, Bihar*)

Target High Hybrid book is a broad spectrum of literary work!
Hybrid features of this book are all the important points, high yield topics, previous year papers and much more for you to level up for your exams. It has explained everything in a broad manner to remove complexity for you. Amazing book overall!"

Kana Ram Maurya (Nawa, Rajasthan)

Download the App Nursing Next Live

Access TARGET HIGH Digital Lite

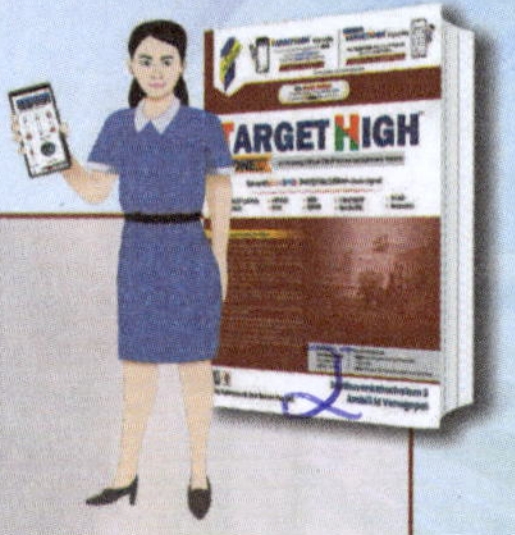

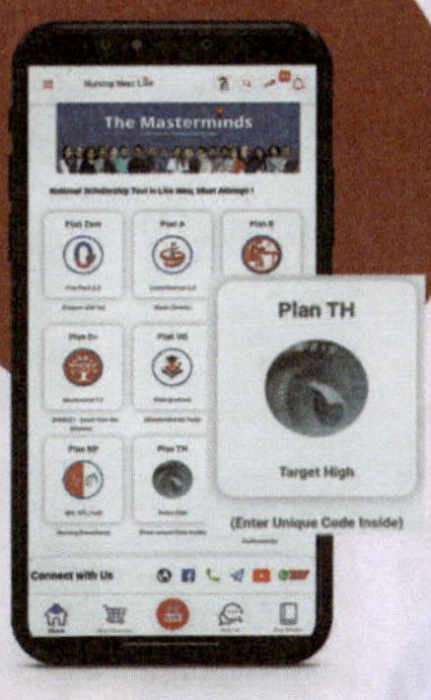

Bridging the Gap Between Theory & Practice through

Conceptual & Animated Videos

200+

Conceptual Videos on Important Topics in Infographic Form with voice-over for easy learning

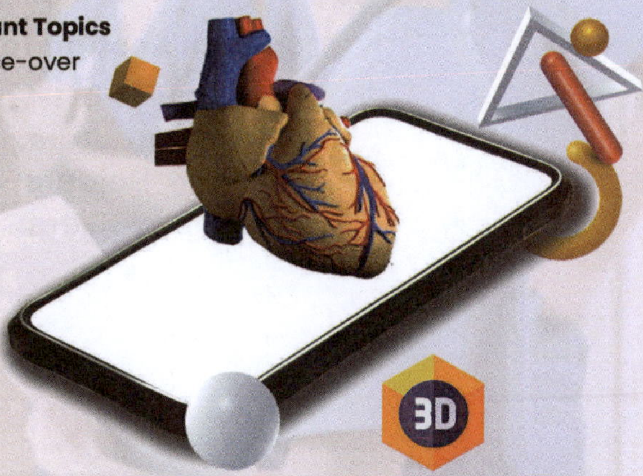

5

3D Animated videos with their descriptions

1. *Positions & Presentations of fetus during labor*
2. *Parts and Diameter of fetal skull*
3. *Body planes & movement*
4. *Respiration: Exchange of gases*
5. *Anatomy of Heart & Cardiac Cycle*

Clinical Learning

It's time to explore the advanced level learning!!

400+	**50+**	**1000+**
Image-Based Questions	**Video-Based Questions**	**Clinical Case-based Questions**

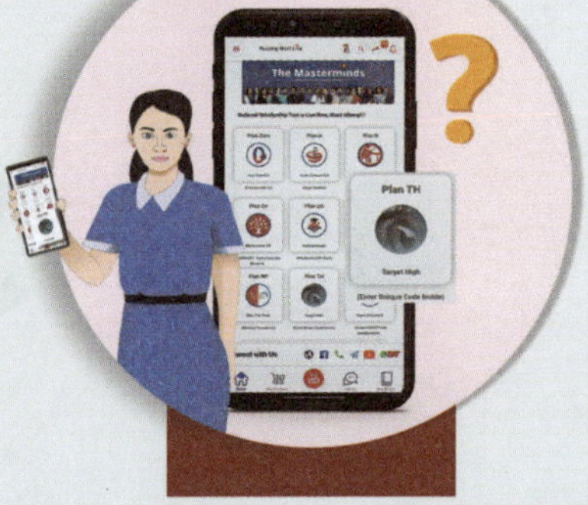

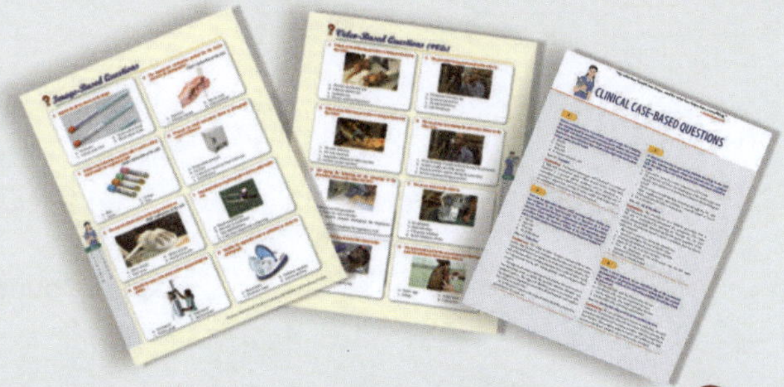

Target High Digital Lite – Best companion for Nursing Aspirants!
This book has proved to be the best preparation companion for any and all nursing exams. Target High Digital Lite has updated new features like chapter-wise and subject-wise clinical based MCQs and the clinical highlights between the synopses, which make reading & practicing MCQs more interesting. This book will always keep you updated.
Zahoor Ahmad Shaikh (Kulgam, J & K)

Target High Hybrid Digital edition: Dil Maange More!
I am much of a book reader but once I started studying the Hybrid features of Target High, I could feel the difference. It has described every single topic and subject in a very precise and intricate manner that made my study quite comprehensive for me. Highly recommended for all.
Shafat Ahmad Naikoo (Pulwama, J & K)

Download the App Nursing Next Live | Access **TARGET HIGH** Digital Lite

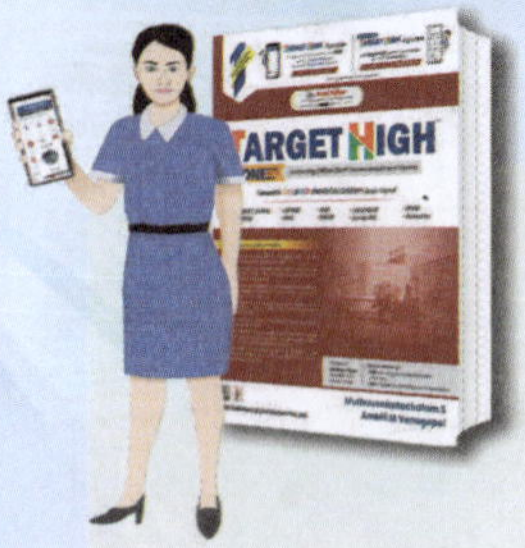

Be in Spotlight

Claim Your Moment: Flourish in the Spotlight by Sharing your success story and feedback

Special Section for

Reviewers
Contributors
Rank Holders
Happy Users

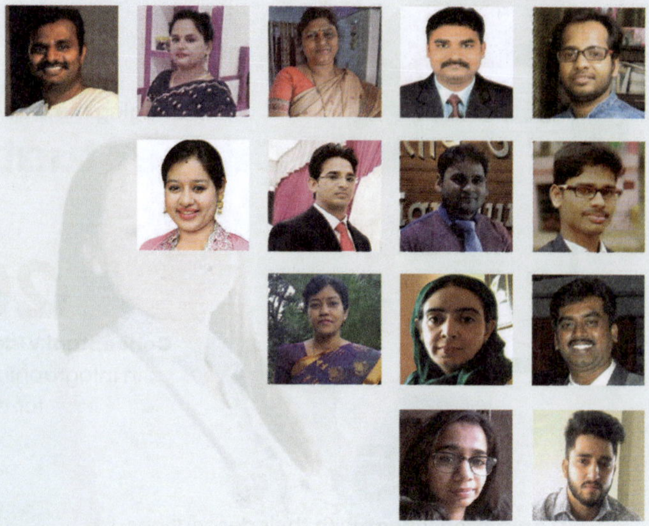

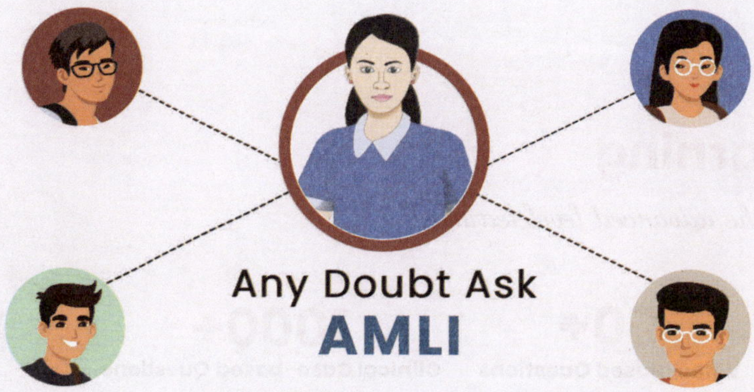

Get your

TARGET HIGH

Queries Resolved from

AMLI (The **TH** Educator)

FROM DOUBTS TO CONFIDENCE

Expert Counseling & Guidance for NORCET Exam

Target High played a vital role in my preparations especially Golden Points

"This book has played an important role in my preparations. I could prepare with all the given features that are listen and recall, assess yourself by tests, etc. You should definitely go for it."

Kana Ram Chotiya *(Jayal, Rajasthan)*

Target High with Updated Features – HIGHLY RECOMMENDED FOR ALL

The content of the Target High Book is excellent and adequate. The target high digital lite has new updated features like "Assess Yourself" in which chapter-wise and subject-wise MCQs are available which will help you to gain confidence in single subject and help you to achieve your ultimate goal.

Shobha Kumari *(Ranchi, Jharkhand)*

TARGET HIGH™

ONE NATION NORCET BOOK on Nursing Officer/Staff Nurse Recruitment Exams

*Not to be sold separately, **FREE** with Target High Seventh Colored Phygital Edition*

***ADD ON Booklet** Focusing on General Knowledge and Aptitude*

Authors

Muthuvenkatachalam Srinivasan
PhD (INC Consortium), MSc Nursing (AIIMS Delhi), D Pharm
RN (NMBA Australia)
Assistant Professor
Institute of Human Behaviour and Allied Sciences (IHBAS)
Govt. of NCT
New Delhi

Ambili M Venugopal
MSc Pediatric Nursing (AIIMS), BSc (Hons) Nursing (AIIMS)
Tutor/Clinical Instructor
College of Nursing
All India Institute of Medical Sciences
Mangalagiri, Andhra Pradesh

Foreword

Roy K George
Sandhya Gupta
Reddemma K
Indarjit Walia

Recommended By

- Usha Ukande
- Ratna Prakash
- Sandhya Ghai
- B V Kathyayni
- Indarjit Walia
- Sabina Ali
- Harinder Jeet Goyal
- B Valli
- Jeyaseelan M Devadason
- Prema P
- Rashmi E John
- T Samuel Ravi
- Shyamala D Manivannan
- Sr Rojamma
- Jacintha D'Souza
- HC Rawat
- Jyoti Sarin
- Sunita Lawrence
- Deepika C Khakha
- Sr Mary Lucita
- L Gopichandran
- Radha Saini
- Saumya Srivastava

CBSPD *Dedicated to Education*

Nursing Knowledge Tree

CBS Publishers & Distributors Pvt Ltd

• New Delhi • Bengaluru • Chennai • Kochi • Kolkata • Lucknow
• Mumbai • Hyderabad • Nagpur • Patna • Pune • Vijayawada

TRADEMARK

Target High is now a registered trademark title of CBS Publishers and Distributors Pvt Ltd and all rights are reserved with the publisher. You are prohibited to use Target High name in any form (book, Facebook page, coaching institute, etc.). Kindly note, the affiliations of the authors are mentioned at the back cover and they don't run any coaching institute with the name Target High. Also, there is only one registered Facebook page of Target High by CBS Publishers and Distributors Pvt Ltd. Any other Facebook page, book or coaching institute are not connected with us.

DISCLAIMER

Target High is a reference title and not a standard resource of information. Careful efforts have been invested in compiling/editing of the concerned data/information given in this book in various sections. However, it is likely that some errors might have crept in despite being vigilant. In such a case, please refer to standard publications for verification, and authors and publishers would not be held responsible in case any of the readers attempts a wrong answer in any of his/her examinations. We are grateful to the authors of the standard textbooks that have been referred to while compiling the text of the book. Questions given in the book are memory based and we do not claim that they are the originally asked questions in examinations. Any such similarity would be purely coincidental.

SET ISBN: 978-93-94525-20-7

Published by **Satish Kumar Jain** and produced by **Varun Jain** for

CBS Publishers & Distributors Pvt Ltd
4819/XI Prahlad Street, 24 Ansari Road, Daryaganj, New Delhi 110 002, India.
Ph: +91-11-23289259, 23266861, 23266867 Website: www.cbspd.com
Fax: 011-23243014
e-mail: delhi@cbspd.com; cbspubs@airtelmail.in.

Corporate Office: 204 FIE, Industrial Area, Patparganj, Delhi 110 092
Ph: +91-11-4934 4934 Fax: 4934 4935
e-mail: feedback@cbspd.com; bhupesharora@cbspd.com

Branches

- **Bengaluru:** Seema House 2975, 17th Cross, K.R. Road, Banasankari 2nd Stage, Bengaluru-560 070, Karnataka
  Ph: +91-80-26771678/79 Fax: +91-80-26771680 e-mail: bangalore@cbspd.com
- **Chennai:** 7, Subbaraya Street, Shenoy Nagar, Chennai-600 030, Tamil Nadu
  Ph: +91-44-26680620, 26681266 Fax: +91-44-42032115 e-mail: chennai@cbspd.com
- **Kochi:** 68/1534, 35, 36-Power House Road, Opp. KSEB, Cochin-682018, Kochi, Kerala
  Ph: +91-484-4059061-65 Fax: +91-484-4059065 e-mail: kochi@cbspd.com
- **Kolkata:** Hind Ceramics Compound, 1st Floor, 147, Nilganj Road, Belghoria, Kolkata-700056, West Bengal
  Ph: +033-2563-3055/56 e-mail: kolkata@cbspd.com
- **Lucknow:** Basement, Khushnuma Complex, 7-Meerabai Marg (Behind Jawahar Bhawan), Lucknow-226001, Uttar Pradesh
  Ph: +0522-4000032 e-mail: tiwari.lucknow@cbspd.com
- **Mumbai:** PWD Shed, Gala No. 25/26, Ramchandra Bhatt Marg, Next to J.J. Hospital Gate No. 2, Opp. Union Bank of India, Noor Baug, Mumbai-400009, Maharashtra
  Ph: +91-22-66661880/89 Fax: +91-22-24902342 e-mail: mumbai@cbspd.com

Representatives

- **Hyderabad** +91-9885175004
- **Pune** +91-9623451994
- **Patna** +91-9334159340
- **Vijayawada** +91-9000660880

Printed at : Goyal Offset Works Pvt. Ltd. Haryana (INDIA)

Booklet Contents

SECTION A What All You Will Get in Target High Digital Lite

SECTION B General Knowledge and Aptitude

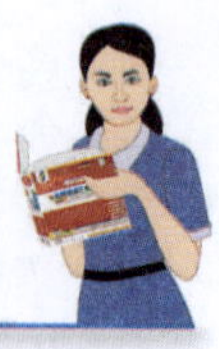

Section A

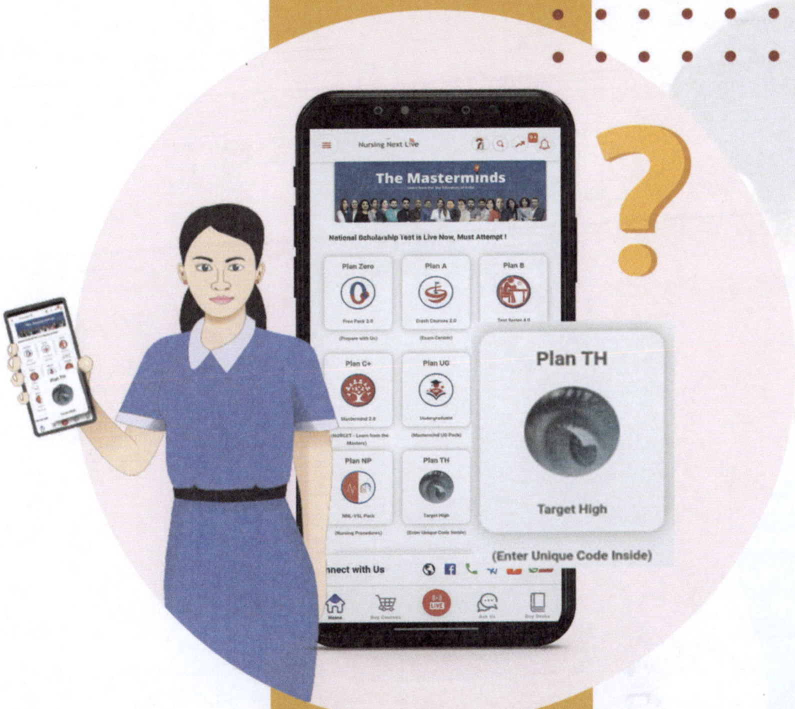

WHAT ALL YOU WILL GET IN TARGET HIGH DIGITAL LITE

- Golden Points
- Assess Yourself
- High Yield Topics
- Previous Year Papers
- Appendices
- 7+ Study Plans
- Conceptual Videos (New Feature)
- Any Doubt, Ask AMLI
- Current Affairs & Aptitude
- Clinical Learning
- Be in Spotlight
- Recent Updates
- 3D Animated Videos

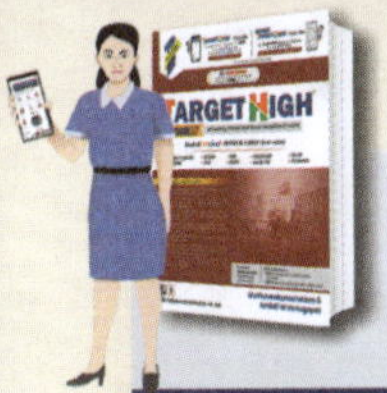

What is PHYGITAL (Physical Book + Digital App)

- Digitalization has changed the whole education system. The technology has altered the common traditional approach of teaching-learning to web-based digital learning. Now anyone can learn anything anytime & anywhere.
- To make your study more interactive with learning materials (Books) we have come-up with PHYGITAL edition of the books. And in the series, our Best Seller Title **Target High** is available in the PHYGITAL edition.
- This hybrid learning is basically a blended learning where in printed books are thoughtfully integrated with digital support to re-conceptualize the learning method in more interactive manner with added values to your knowledge.
- It provides you flexibility of learning; the option of freedom to study theoretical concept with books and enhancement of skills through practically learning on digitally interactive support.
- Target High PHYGITAL Edition in an endeavor to give you the next level preparation for any nursing competitive exams, where you can do More Practice, More Learning through Audio-Visual aids, More number of Tests, Plenty of Quality-content, lots of flexibility, Customization and engaging-interactive learning experiences with its digital support **"TARGET HIGH DIGITAL lite"**.

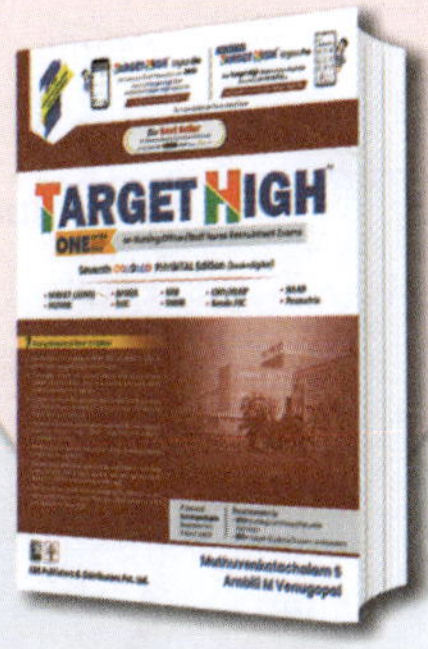

HOW TARGET HIGH PHYGITAL EDITION WILL HELP YOU IN PREPARATION?

- Helps in both, developing and understanding concepts from the book & practical application of concept with **Digital Support**
- Keeps you updated from all the recent advances & up to date content time to time.
- Provides flexibility to access the important content anytime anywhere, you can learn and practice at your move
- You can access to both Book content & Recent Updates added regularly in the **PHYGITAL** edition
- You can read from the Book & Watch, Listen & Practice on the digital support – **TH Digital Lite**
- Imparts Audio - Visual aids to the learning with the loaded Podcast and Videos
- Provides 24-hours of learning resource and assistance for your any doubts and queries from the book as well from its digital support
- Provides additional content with each monthly updates which is not covered in book to maintain consistency in your learning and flow of knowledge
- Generates a daily habit of attempting and practicing the tests on digital platform along with the **National level ranking** for your assessment
- Analyses and assists in identifying your strength and weakness to improve your efficiency with complete coverage of new INC Syllabus
- Educate yourself with TH Digital educator, AMLI who guides you at each single step of preparation and learning

8 AMAZING FEATURES OF TARGET HIGH DIGITAL LITE

- **GOLDEN POINTS** Listen & Recall: 3000+ Golden Points in Podcast Format covering all Subjects.
- **ASSESS YOURSELF** Read and Practice: 80+ Subject-wise tests covering 7500+ Qs of all Subjects, and 48 Grand Tests covering 4800 Qs focusing NORCET 6.0 and 7.0.
- **HIGH YIELD TOPICS** Revise on the Go: 300+ High Yield Topics (Tables + Images) for quick access.
- **ADD Ons** Dil Mange More Content: 115+ Previous Year Papers (20 Papers with their Rationale and 90+ without Rationale), 75+ Appendices, Monthly Current Affairs, Recent Updates, 20 Nursing Skill Procedures, How to Prepare for Staff Competitive Exams, How to Appear in the Interview for Nursing Tutor, and Study Planner for AIIMS NORCET Exams with Tips and Tricks, Decoding the Case Scenario-Based Questions, How to Prepare for NORCET Stage I-Prelims and NORCET Stage II-Mains: An overview and plenty of ADD-ON content.
- **CLINICAL LEARNING:** 400+ Image-Based Qs, 50+ Video-Based Qs and 1000+ Clinical Case-Based Qs
- **CONCEPTUAL & ANIMATED VIDEOS:** 200+ Important Topics Conceptual Videos in Infographic Form with voice-over for easy learning and **5** 3-D Animated videos with their description
  - Position & Presentations of fetus during labor
  - Parts and Diameter of fetal skull
  - Body planes & movement
  - Respiration: Exchange of gases
  - Anatomy of Heart & Cardiac Cycle
- **Any Doubt? Ask AMLI!:** Get your Target High queries resolved by AMLI, your Target High Virtual Educator.
- **Be in SPOTLIGHT:** Special Section for Contributors/Reviewers/ Rank Holders and Happy Users. Share your success stories and feedback and get featured in the book.

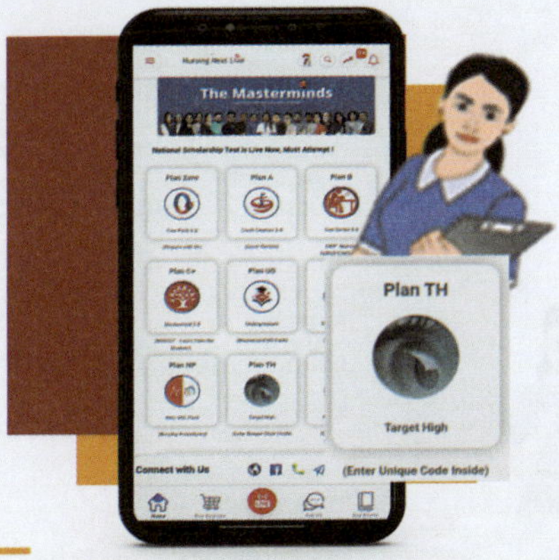

1 GOLDEN POINTS

3000+ Golden Points with Voice-Over (Pre-loaded & Forthcoming)

S. No.	Subjects	No's	
1.	Fundamentals of Nursing	100	
2.	Medical Surgical Nursing/Adult Health Nursing	660	
3.	Pharmacology	172	
4.	Community Health Nursing	124	
5.	Psychiatric Nursing	252	
6.	Pediatric Nursing	121	
7.	Obstetric and Gynecological Nursing	277	
8.	Applied Microbiology	71	
9.	Applied Biochemistry and Nutrition	118	
10.	Applied Sociology and Psychology	78	
11.	Nursing Research and Statistics	35	
12.	Nursing Education	26	
13.	Nursing Administration and Management	28	
14.	Computer/Health and Nursing Informatics	52	
15.	Forensic Nursing and Indian Laws	36	
16.	Arithmetic and Numerical Ability	350	
17.	Forthcoming Golden Points Based on NORCET 2023 & NORCET 2024	500	Tentative
		3000	

2 ASSESS YOURSELF

8000+ Subject wise MCQs in **90+** Tests (Pre-loaded -7000 MCQs) & 200+ Newly added Exclusive in App + 700 Qs will be covered in Future Updates

S. No.	Subject	Total Qs [Pre-loaded (Book + App)]	Total sets of Test (Based on NORCET)	Newly added (Exclusive in App)
1.	Fundamentals of Nursing	820	10	35
2.	Medical Surgical Nursing/Adult Health Nursing	1060	12	100
3.	Pharmacology	620	8	20
4.	Community Health Nursing	840	10	–
5.	Psychiatric Nursing	820	10	–
6.	Pediatric Nursing	840	10	–
7.	Obstetric and Gynecological Nursing	820	10	20
8.	Applied Microbiology	170	4	–
9.	Applied Biochemistry and Nutrition	200	3	10
10.	Applied Sociology and Psychology	–	–	5
11.	Nursing Research and Statistics	320	5	10
12.	Nursing Education	100	2	–
13.	Nursing Administration and Management	200	2	15

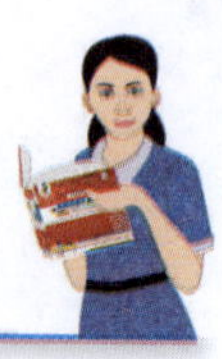

Contd...

S. No.	Subject	Total Qs [Pre-loaded (Book + App)]	Total sets of Test (Based on NORCET)	Newly added (Exclusive in App)
14.	Computer/Health and Nursing Informatics	100	2	–
15.	Forensic Nursing and Indian Laws	–	–	10
16.	GK/English/Aptitude/Arithmetic and Numerical Ability	140	3	–
17.	New MCQs in Future Updates	725	–	–
	Total Qs	8000	91	–

48 Grand Tests (Prelims/Mains) Based on New Exam Pattern covering 4800 Qs based on Target High 7/e Edition for Practice

Grand Tests				
Test No	**Date**	**Test Type**	**No. of Sets**	**No. of Qs**
1.	20th September 2023	NORCET Mains	1	100
2.	30th September 2023	NORCET Mains	1	100
3.	15th October 2023	NORCET Prelims	1	100
4.	30th October 2023	NORCET Mains	1	100
5.	15th November 2023	NORCET Prelims	1	100
6.	30th November 2023	NORCET Mains	1	100
7.	15th December 2023	NORCET Prelims	1	100
8.	30th December 2023	NORCET Mains	1	100
9.	15th January 2024	NORCET Prelims	1	100
10.	30th January 2024	NORCET Mains	1	100
11.	15th February 2024	NORCET Prelims	1	100
12.	30th February 2024	NORCET Mains	1	100
13.	15th March 2024	NORCET Prelims	1	100
14.	30th March 2024	NORCET Mains	1	100
15.	15th April 2024	NORCET Prelims	1	100
16.	30th April 2024	NORCET Mains	1	100
17.	15th May 2024	NORCET Prelims	1	100
18.	30th May 2024	NORCET Mains	1	100
19.	15th June 2024	NORCET Prelims	1	100
20.	30th June 2024	NORCET Mains	1	100
21.	15th July 2024	NORCET Prelims	1	100
22.	30th July 2024	NORCET Mains	1	100
23.	15th August 2024	NORCET Prelims	1	100
24.	30th August 2024	NORCET Mains	1	100
25.	15th September 2024	NORCET Prelims	1	100
26.	30th September 2024	NORCET Mains	1	100
27.	15th October 2024	NORCET Prelims	1	100
28.	30th October 2024	NORCET Mains	1	100
29.	15th November 2024	NORCET Prelims	1	100
30.	30th November 2024	NORCET Mains	1	100
31.	15th December 2024	NORCET Prelims	1	100

Contd...

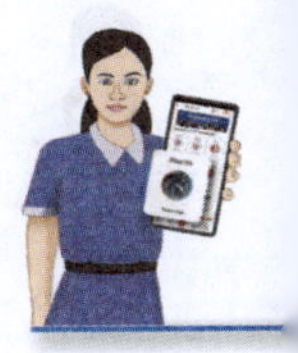

What All You Will Get in Target High Digital Lite

Grand Tests				
Test No	**Date**	**Test Type**	**No. of Sets**	**No. of Qs**
32.	30th December 2024	NORCET Mains	1	100
33.	15th January 2025	NORCET Prelims	1	100
34.	30th January 2025	NORCET Mains	1	100
35.	15th February 2025	NORCET Prelims	1	100
36.	30th February 2025	NORCET Mains	1	100
37.	15th March 2025	NORCET Prelims	1	100
38.	30th March 2025	NORCET Mains	1	100
39.	15th April 2025	NORCET Prelims	1	100
40.	30th April 2025	NORCET Mains	1	100
41.	15th May 2025	NORCET Prelims	1	100
42.	30th May 2025	NORCET Mains	1	100
43.	15th June 2025	NORCET Prelims	1	100
44.	30th June 2025	NORCET Mains	1	100
45.	15th July 2025	NORCET Prelims	1	100
46.	30th July 2025	NORCET Mains	1	100
47.	15th August 2025	NORCET Prelims	1	100
48.	30th August 2025	NORCET Mains	1	100

The test type is based on the current and future NORCET exam pattern. In future, if the exam pattern changes then accordingly the Grand Test pattern will also be changed without any prior information.

20 Special Tests (NORCET pattern) covering 200 Qs each – Total Qs 4000

Special Test			
Set No.	**Test**	**Topic**	**No. of Qs**
Set 1	TH Special Test-1	Pattern of NORCET 2023 (June)	200
Set 2	TH Special Test-2	Pattern of NORCET 2023 (June)	200
Set 3	TH Special Test-3	Pattern of NORCET 2023 (June)	200
Set 4	TH Special Test-4	Pattern of NORCET 2023 (June)	200
Set 5	TH Special Test-5	Pattern of NORCET 2023 (June)	200
Set 6	TH Special Test-6	Pattern of NORCET 2023 (June)	200
Set 7	TH Special Test-7	Pattern of NORCET 2023 (June)	200
Set 8	TH Special Test-8	Pattern of NORCET 2023 (June)	200
Set 9	TH Special Test-9	Pattern of NORCET 2023 (June)	200
Set 10	TH Special Test-10	Pattern of NORCET 2023 (June)	200
Set 11	TH Special Test-11	Pattern of NORCET 2023 (June)	200
Set 12	TH Special Test-12	Pattern of NORCET 2023 (June)	200
Set 13	TH Special Test-13	Pattern of NORCET 2023 (June)	200
Set 14	TH Special Test-14	Pattern of NORCET 2023 (June)	200
Set 15	TH Special Test-15	Pattern of NORCET 2023 (June)	200
Set 16	TH Special Test-16	Pattern of NORCET 2023 (June)	200
Set 17	TH Special Test-17	Pattern of NORCET 2023 (June)	200
Set 18	TH Special Test-18	Pattern of NORCET 2023 (June)	200
Set 19	TH Special Test-19	Pattern of NORCET 2023 (June)	200
Set 20	TH Special Test-20	Pattern of NORCET 2023 (June)	200

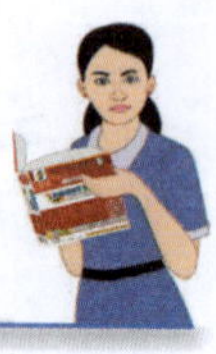

All the TH Special tests are based on the Pattern of NORCET 2023 (June) with National Level Ranking

What All You Will Get in Target High Digital Lite

3 HIGH YIELD TOPICS

300+ High Yield Tables & Images covered with detailed description (Pre-loaded & Forthcoming)

S. No.	Subject	Total Quantity	Tables	Images
1.	Fundamentals of Nursing	24	12	12
2.	Medical Surgical Nursing/Adult Health Nursing	34	8	26
3.	Pharmacology	13	13	–
4.	Community Health Nursing	24	13	11
5.	Psychiatric Nursing	21	17	4
6.	Pediatric Nursing	18	9	9
7.	Obstetric and Gynecological Nursing	30	8	22
8.	Applied Microbiology	6	5	1
9.	Applied Biochemistry and Nutrition	7	5	2
10.	Nursing Research and Statistics	10	3	7
11.	Nursing Education	9	6	3
12.	Nursing Administration and Management	2	1	1
13.	Computer/Health and Nursing Informatics	5	5	–
14.	Newly added in various subjects (Forthcoming-Forensic Nursing and Indian Laws, Applied Sociology and Psychology, etc.)	100	–	–
	Total Tables & Images	303		

4 PREVIOUS YEAR PAPERS

115+ Previous Year Papers of National & State level exams, covering 2023–2004 (Selected Papers are with Rationale)

New (Previous Year Papers)

1.	NORCET 2023
2.	AIIMS Jodhpur (Senior Nursing Officer) 2023
3.	AIIMS Bibinagar (Tutor) 2023
4.	AIIMS Bibinagar Associate Professor 2023
5.	Sree Chitra Tirunal Institute for Medical Science and Technology (Nursing Officer) 2023
6.	Uttar Pradesh University of Medical Sciences (Nursing Officer) 2023
7.	NORCET (Nursing Officer) 2022 (Memory-based)
8.	Staff Nurse Examination Himachal Pradesh (October 2022)
9.	Western Coalfields Limited 2022
10.	Odisha Sub-Ordinate Staff Selection Commission 2022
11.	Nursing Officer/Principal, Gujarat Nursing Service 2022
12.	NORCET (Nursing Officer) 2021 (Memory-based)

Pre-loaded

Papers in Nursing Next Live App (Under Target High Digital Lite)

1.	AIIMS NORCET 2022 Recall (Shift 1)
2.	AIIMS NORCET 2021 (Shift 1) Recall (with rationale)
3.	AIIMS NORCET 2021 (Shift 2) Recall (with rationale)
4.	AIIMS Raipur (Lecturer) 2021

Contd...

5.	AIIMS NORCET 2020 (with rationale)
6.	AIIMS Jodhpur (Nursing Officer) 2020 (with rationale)
7.	AIIMS Nagpur (Nursing Officer) 2020
8.	AIIMS Patna (Nursing Officer) 2020

Contd...

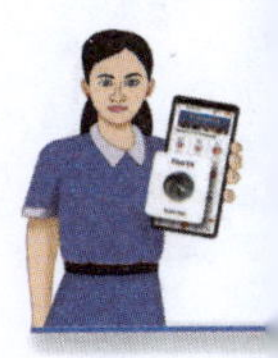

9.	AIIMS Raipur (Nursing Officer) 2019
10.	AIIMS Bathinda (Nursing Officer) 2019
11.	AIIMS Raipur (Nursing Officer) 2019; Shift 1
12.	AIIMS Raipur (Nursing Officer) 2019; Shift 2
13.	AIIMS Raipur (Nursing Officer) 2019; Shift 3
14.	AIIMS Bhubaneswar (Senior Nursing Officer) 2019
15.	AIIMS New Delhi (Nursing Officer) 2019
16.	AIIMS New Delhi (Nursing Officer) 2018
17.	AIIMS Nagpur (Nursing Officer) 2018
18.	AIIMS Jodhpur (Senior Nursing Officer) Grade 1: 2018
19.	AIIMS Bhopal (Senior Nursing Officer) 2018
20.	AIIMS Bhopal (Nursing Officer) 2018; Shift 1
21.	AIIMS Bhopal (Nursing Officer) 2018; Shift 2
22.	AIIMS Mangalagiri (Nursing Officer) Grade-II; 2018; Shift 2
23.	AIIMS Bhubaneswar (Nursing Officer) 2018
24.	AIIMS Raipur (Nursing Officer) 2017; Shift 1
25.	AIIMS Raipur (Nursing Officer) 2017; Shift 2
26.	AIIMS Raipur (Nursing Officer) 2017; Shift 3
27.	AIIMS Raipur (Nursing Tutor) 2017
28.	AIIMS Jodhpur & Rishikesh (Nursing Officer) 2017
29.	AIIMS Raipur (Senior Nursing Officer) 2017
30.	AIIMS Bhopal (Nursing Officer) 2016
31.	AIIMS New Delhi (Nursing Officer) 2016
32.	AIIMS Bhopal (Senior Nursing Officer) 2016
33.	CNCI (Nursing Officer) 2021
34.	BFUHS 2021
35.	ESIC Paramedical 2019; Shift 1
36.	ESIC Paramedical 2019; Shift 2
37.	ESIC (Nursing Officer) 2016; Shift 1
38.	ESIC (Nursing Officer) 2016; Shift 2
39.	ESIC (Nursing Officer) Bangalore Shift 1: 2016
40.	ESIC (Nursing Officer) Bangalore Shift 2: 2016
41.	ESIC (Nursing Officer) Delhi 2016
42.	ESIC (Nursing Officer) Bangalore 2013
43.	ESIC (Nursing Officer) Chennai 2012
44.	ESIC (Nursing Officer) Grade II: 20
45.	ESIC (Nursing Officer) Ahmedabad 2011
46.	Kerala PSC 2021 (with rationale)
47.	Kerala PSC (Nursing Officer) 2017
48.	Kerala PSC (Nursing Officer) 2016
49.	Kerala PSC (Nursing Officer) 2014
50.	Kerala PSC (Nursing Officer) Grade II: 2011
51.	Kerala PSC (Nursing Officer) Set C: 2011
52.	Kerala PSC (Nursing Officer) 2010
53.	BHU (Nursing Officer) 2019

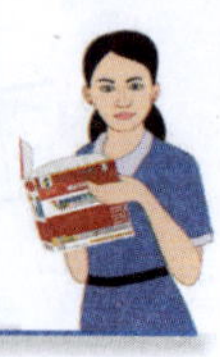

Contd...

54.	BHU (Nursing Officer) 2018
55.	BHU (Nursing Officer) 2016
56.	BHU (Nursing Officer) 2015
57.	Safdarjung (Nursing Officer) 2019
58.	Safdarjung (Nursing Officer) 2018
59.	JIPMER (Nursing Officer) 2020
60.	JIPMER (Nursing Officer) 2013
61.	JIPMER (Nursing Officer) 2012
62.	UK State MSc (Nursing Officer) 2016
63.	UK Nursing Tutor (Paper 1- Set B)
64.	RRB (Nursing Officer) 2019; Shift 1 (with rationale)
65.	RRB (Nursing Officer) 2019; Shift 2
66.	RRB (Nursing Officer) 2019; Shift 3
67.	RRB (Nursing Officer) 2019; Shift 4
68.	RRB (Nursing Officer) 2019; Shift 5
69.	RRB Paramedical PHN 2015
70.	RRB (Nursing Officer) 2015; Set A
71.	RRB (Nursing Officer) 2015; Set B
72.	RRB (Nursing Officer) 2015; Set C
73.	RRB Secunderabad (Senior Nursing Officer) 2015
74.	RRB (Nursing Officer) 2012
75.	HPSSC (Nursing Officer) 2016
76.	HP (Nursing Officer) 2016
77.	RAK MSc Entrance Exam 2018
78.	RAK New Delhi Entrance Exam 2017
79.	GMCH (Nursing Officer) 2019
80.	GMCH (Nursing Officer) 2016
81.	Daman and Diu (Nursing Officer) 2018
82.	Northern Coal Field Limited, Singrauli (Nursing Officer) 2019
83.	PGIMER Chandigarh (Nursing Officer) 2016
84.	CHO Haryana 2021
85.	CHO Rajasthan 2020
86.	CHO Madhya Pradesh 2020
87.	CHO Madhya Pradesh 2019 Shift-1
88.	CHO Uttar Pradesh 2018
89.	RUHS MSc Nursing Entrance Exam 2018
90.	RUHS MSc Nursing Entrance Exam 2016
91.	RUHS Post Basic Nursing Entrance Exam 2016
92.	LNJP Hospital Delhi (Nursing Officer) 2012
93.	DSSSB Shift I (NO) 2019
94.	DSSSB Shift II (NO) 2019
95.	DSSSB PHN 2015
96.	DSSSB ANM 2015
97.	Jhalawar Hospital and Medical College Society 2012

Contd...

98.	TNPSC Maternal and Child Health Officer 2015	103.	Rohtak (Nursing Officer) 2020
99.	RML Hospital (Nursing Officer) 2011	104.	NIMHANS (Nursing Officer) 2019
100.	Insurance Medical Services (Nursing Officer) 2004	105.	SKIM (Nursing Officer) 2020 Paper (New)
101.	RRC (Nursing Officer) 2012	106.	Gujarat Staff (Nursing Officer) 2021 (New)
102.	SCTIMST (Nursing Officer) 2015	107.	Jr. Grade Nurse/Jr. Staff Nurse/Jr. Nurse 2020

What All You Will Get in Target High Digital Lite

5 APPENDICES

S. No.	Topic	Sub-topic
1.	Anatomy and Physiology	1. Blood supply of heart 2. Lobes of brain and their functions 3. Quadrants of abdomen 4. Cranial nerves, their types and functions 5. Types of joints in human body 6. Functions of sympathetic and parasympathetic nervous system 7. Fetal skull 8. Fetal circulation and its postnatal changes
2.	All about COVID-19	1. Updates on COVID-19 2. Management of COVID-19 in pregnancy 3. Mucormycosis (black fungus) 4. Updated questions on COVID-19 5. Sequence of donning and doffing of PPE while caring for COVID-19 Patients
3.	Instruments and Equipment	1. Instruments 2. Equipment/Instruments 3. Obstetrics and Gynecological instruments 4. Tubes and Catheters 5. Decontamination of equipment and unit 6. Slings and splints 7. Cold chain methods and equipment
4.	Positions and Presentations	1. Positions 2. Positions and presentations of fetus during Labor
5.	Program, Policies and Recent Updates	1. Recent updates on community health nursing 2. Norms for health personnel/centers in community 3. Demography in India 4. Review of health programs in India, launch year and objectives 5. Health planning in India 6. Some Important Social Welfare/Health/Development Program Launched by Government of India from August 2014 till April 2021. 7. Community nutrition program 8. Immunization schedule 9. Color coding for medical gas cylinders 10. Biomedical waste management rules 2016 11. Some important social welfare/health/development program launched by government of India from August 2014 till June 2023 (new)
6.	Disease Conditions	1. Updates on tuberculosis 2. Some disease conditions and their primary signs/symptoms 3. Communicable diseases 4. Vitamins: functions, sources and deficiency diseases
7.	Assessment, Prevention and Management	1. Frye's ABCDE cascade for prioritizing centre 2. Glasgow coma scale 3. Triage categories 4. Arterial blood gas 5. Shocks- types, managements and solutions

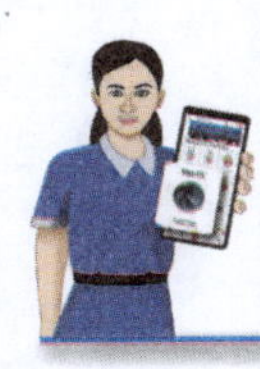

Contd...

S. No.	Topic	Sub-topic
		6. Skeletal and skin traction 7. ECG waveforms and pathological findings 8. Common scales used for assessment/treatment 9. Level of spinal cord injury and associated motor loss 10. Neurotransmitters chart 11. Interpretation of BMI 12. Acute coronary syndromes and their treatments 13. Level of prevention 14. Vaccines used to prevent diseases 15. Classification of mental retardation 16. EGO defence mechanisms with examples 17. Phases of wound healing process 18. Phobias 19. Blood groups 20. Burns 21. Radiating pain/referred pain 22. Endocrine glands and hormones 23. Leopold's maneuver
8.	Pharmacology	1. Specific antidotes against poisoning 2. Drug storage and temperature 3. Drugs and their actions 4. Types of insulin 5. Immunoglobulins and their characteristics
9.	Abbreviations	1. Abbreviations
10.	Measurement and Values	1. Conversion from Celsius (°C) to Fahrenheit (°F) 2. Normal values 3. Lung volumes and capacities
11.	Growth and Development	1. Growth and development 2. Comparison of components for adults, children and infants BLS/CPR 3. Stages of personality development
12.	Acts and Legislation	1. Acts and legislations

6 7+ STUDY PLANS

S. No.	Topic
1.	How to Prepare for NORCET 6.0 from TH
2.	How to Prepare for NORCET 7.0 from TH
3.	How to Refer TH while you are in UG
4.	New Informative Blogs
5.	How to Crack CBT Examination
6.	How to Prepare for an Interview
7.	How to Use Target High Lite 7/e – New Approach New Concept

7 CONCEPTUAL VIDEOS (NEW FEATURE)

200+ Important topics conceptual videos in infographic form – **Forthcoming – Detailed list will be uploaded in the App**

8 ANY DOUBT, ASK AMLI

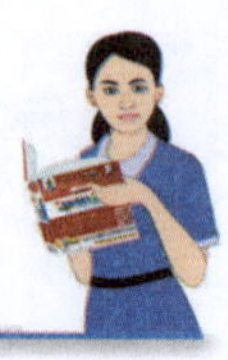

Get all your queries resolved by AMLI within 48 Hrs and also get Guidance Sessions

9 CURRENT AFFAIRS & APTITUDE

100+ Pages E-booklet covering Current Affairs, General Knowledge, General Aptitude along with Practice Qs

What All You Will Get in Target High Digital Lite

10 CLINICAL LEARNING

CBQs, IBQs & VBQS - (350 IBQs & VBQs Pre-loaded) + (620 New CBQs) (64 New IBQs Exclusive in App)

Clinical Case-Based Qs

S. No.	Subject	In Book & App	Exclusive in App	Total
1.	Fundamentals of Nursing	111	22	133
2.	Medical Surgical Nursing/Adult Health Nursing	186	3	189
3.	Pharmacology	–	–	–
4.	Community Health Nursing	–	–	–
5.	Psychiatric Nursing	79	–	79
6.	Pediatric Nursing	104	12	116
7.	Obstetric and Gynecological Nursing	43	60	103
8.	Applied Microbiology	–	–	–
9.	Applied Biochemistry and Nutrition	–	–	–
10.	Applied Sociology and Psychology	–	–	–
11.	Nursing Research and Statistics	–	–	–
12.	Nursing Education	–	–	–
13.	Nursing Administration and Management	–	–	–
14.	Computer/Health and Nursing Informatics	–	–	–
15.	Forensic Nursing and Indian Laws	–	–	–
16.	Anatomy and Phsyiology	–	–	–
17.	GK/English/Aptitude/Arithmetic and Numerical Ability	–	–	–
	Total Qs	523	97	620

IBQS & VBQS

S. No.	Subject	Total Qs	IBQs [Pre-loaded (Book + App)]	New IBQs (Exclusive in App)	VBQs
1.	Fundamentals of Nursing	81	60	3	18
2.	Medical Surgical Nursing/Adult Health Nursing	109	60	26	23
3.	Pharmacology	14	12	2	–
4.	Community Health Nursing	36	32	4	–
5.	Psychiatric Nursing	26	23	3	–
6.	Pediatric Nursing	49	40	3	6
7.	Obstetric and Gynecological Nursing	73	50	17	6
8.	Applied Microbiology	28	26	2	–
9.	Applied Biochemistry and Nutrition	10	10		–
10.	Applied Sociology and Psychology	–	–	–	–
11.	Nursing Research and Statistics	1	–	1	–
12.	Nursing Education	3	–	3	–
13.	Nursing Administration and Management	–	–	–	–
14.	Computer/Health and Nursing Informatics	–	–	–	–
15.	Forensic Nursing and Indian Laws	–	–	–	–
16.	Anatomy & Physiology	18	18	–	–
17.	GK/English/Aptitude/Arithmetic and Numerical Ability	22	22	–	–
	Total Qs	474	357	64	53

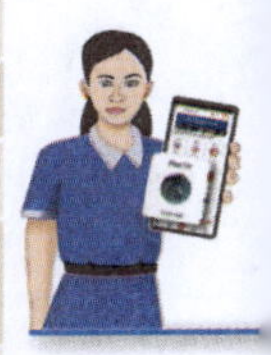

11 BE IN SPOTLIGHT

- **500+** Reviewers' and contributors' details from 22 States & 2 Union Territories (120 Cities from India) - (In Pdf).

12 RECENT UPDATES

NORCET 2023 September & NORCET 2024 (Recall Papers) will be given in Pdf form – Post Examination.

13 3D ANIMATED VIDEOS

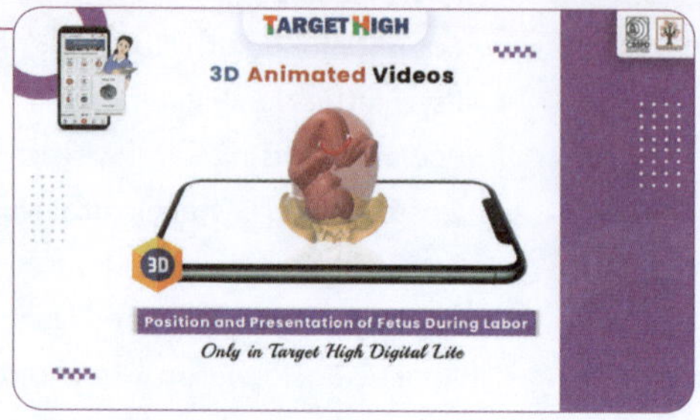

Position and Presentation of Fetus During Labor

The video provides a visual portrayal of the evolving position and presentation of the fetus during different stages of labor. It illustrates how the baby's orientation within the mother's pelvis changes as labor progresses. The video highlights how these positions may impact the birthing process.

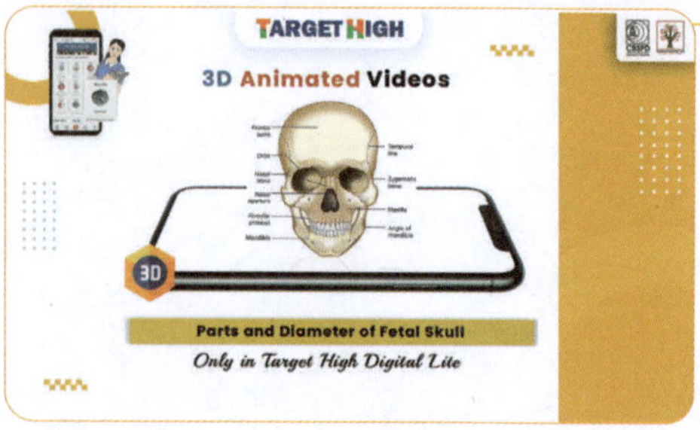

Parts and Diameter of Fetal Skull

The video demonstrates the components and dimensions of the fetal skull, highlighting its dynamic and complex nature. The fetal skull consists of vital parts and diameters crucial for assessing development and facilitating safe childbirth. Fontanelles, soft areas where skull bones have yet to fuse and Sutures, like the sagittal running from front to back and the coronal crossing from ear to ear, permit gentle movement.

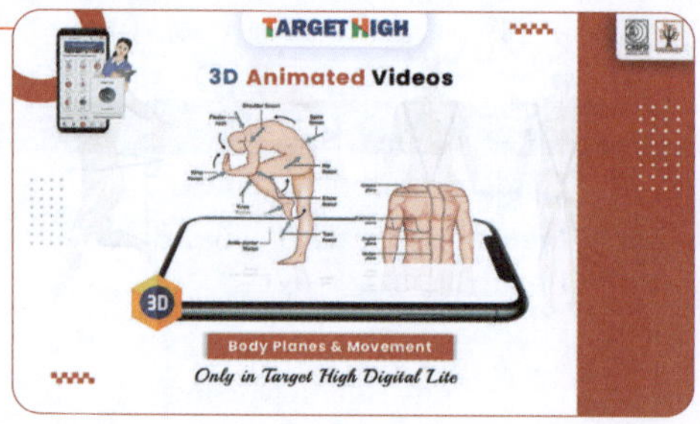

Body Planes and Movement

The video explains the midsagittal, sagittal, coronal or frontal and transverse or horizontal planes of the body along with description of terms related to different body movements like-flexion, extension, adduction, abduction, supination, pronation, etc. to enhance conceptual knowledge related to body movements and anatomical planes.

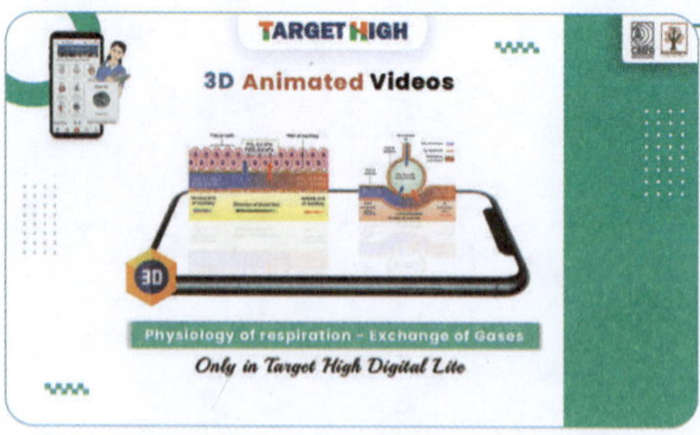

Physiology of Respiration-Exchange of Gases

The video demonstrates the exchange of gases during respiration. Respiration, in the context of living organisms, refers to the process of exchanging gases between an organism and its environment. It involves the intake of oxygen (O_2) and the release of carbon dioxide (CO_2). This is the vital Process for maintaining the proper functioning of cells and sustaining life in various organisms.

Anatomy of Heart and Cardiac Cycle

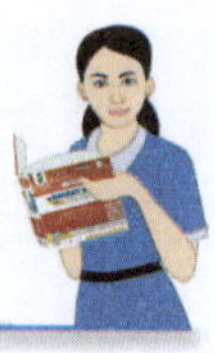

The video demonstrates the external features of heart, chambers of the heart, blood supply, conduction system and electrical events of heart along with conceptual and thorough description of all the events and mechanism of cardiac cycle.

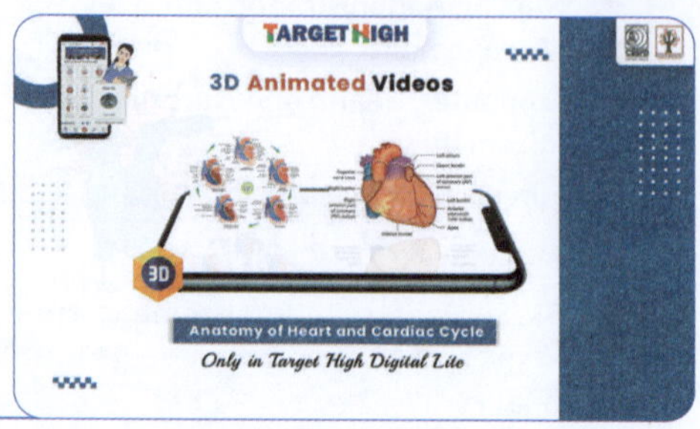

Section B

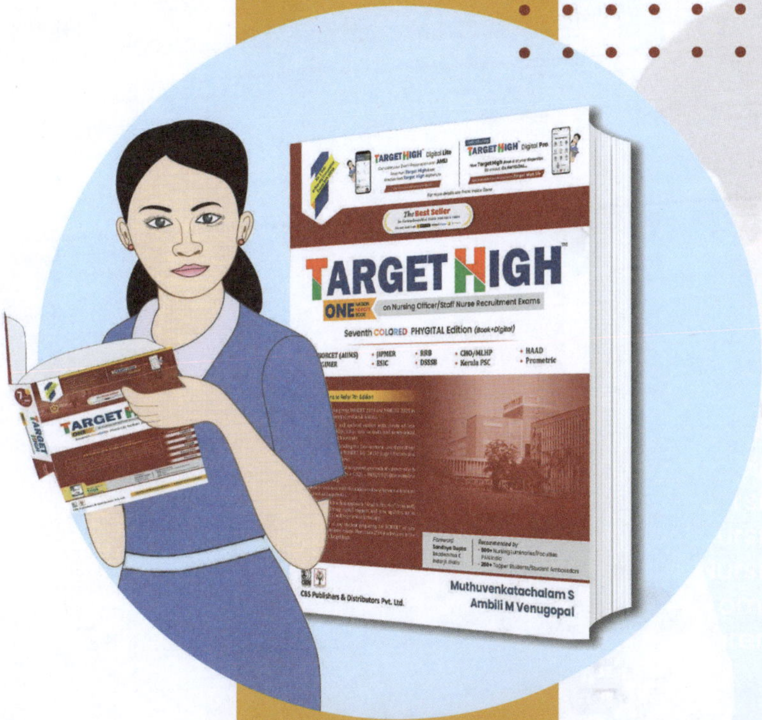

GENERAL KNOWLEDGE AND APTITUDE

- General Knowledge
- General English and Comprehension
- General Intelligence and Reasoning Ability
- Arithmetical and Numerical Ability

"When you are sick of your sickness, you are no longer sick."
—Chinese Proverb

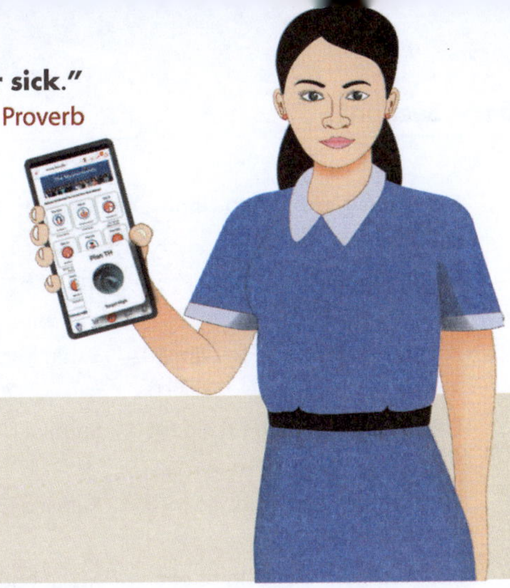

CHAPTER 1

GENERAL KNOWLEDGE

FIRST IN INDIA (MALE)

First Governor of Bengal	Lord Clive
First Governor General of Bengal	Warren Hastings
First Governor General of India	Lord William Bentinck
First Viceroy of India	Lord Canning
First President of Indian National Congress	W. C. Banerjee
First Muslim President of Indian National Congress	Badruddin Tayab Ji
First Governor General of Independent India	Louis Mountbatten
First Indian Governor General of Independent India	C. Rajagopalachari
First Indian to pass ICS Exam	Satyendranath Tagore
First Indian Cosmonaut (to go into space)	Sqn. Ldr. Rakesh Sharma
First Indian Judge of International Court of Justice	Dr Nagendra Nath
First Indian to get Bharat Ratna Award	C. Rajagopalachari, Sarvepalli Radhakrishnan and C. V. Raman
First Indian to swim across the English Channel	Mihir Sen
First Muslim President of India	Dr Zakir Hussain
First Speaker of Lok Sabha	G. V. Mavlankar
First President of Independent India	Dr Rajendra Prasad
First Vice-President of Independent India	Dr S. Radhakrishnan
First Prime Minister of Independent India	Pt. Jawahar Lal Nehru
First Education Minister of Independent India	Maulana Abul Kalam Azad
First person to get Paramvir Chakra	Major Somnath Sharma
First Indian Scientist to get Nobel Prize	C. V. Raman
First Chinese pilgrim to visit India	Fa–Hien
First Minister to resign from Indian Union Cabinet	Shyama Prasad Mukherjee
First British to visit India	John Mildenhall
First Chief Justice of India	Hiralal J Kania

Contd...

FIRST IN INDIA (FEMALE)

First Woman President of India	Pratibha Devi Singh Patil
First Woman Prime Minister of India	Indira Gandhi
First Woman Governor of Indian State	Sarojini Naidu
First Woman Ruler of Delhi Throne	Razia Sultan
First Woman IPS Officer	Kiran Bedi
First Woman Chief Minister of Indian State	Sucheta Kripalani (UP)
First Woman Union Minister	Rajkumari Amrit Kaur
First Woman President of Indian National Congress	Annie Besant
First Woman Judge of Supreme Court	Meera Sahib Fatima Bibi
First Woman to get Ashoka Chakra	Nirja Mishra
First Indian Woman Ambassador at United Nations	Vijayalakshmi Pandit
First Indian Woman to swim across English Channel	Arati Saha Gupta
First Indian Woman to get the Nobel Prize	Mother Teresa
First Indian Woman to climb the Mount Everest	Bachendri Pal
First Indian Woman to become Miss World	Reita Faria
First Indian Woman to become Miss Universe	Sushmita Sen

Contd...

First Indian Woman to climb Mt. Everest twice	Santosh Yadav
First Indian Woman to get Bharat Ratna	Indira Gandhi
First Indian Woman to win WTA Title	Sania Mirza
First Indian Woman president of INC	Sarojini Naidu
First Indian Woman to go into Space	Kalpana Chawla
First Woman Musician to get Bharat Ratna	MS Subbulakshmi
First Woman Chief Justice of High Court	Leela Seth

REVOLUTIONS IN INDIA

Revolution	Field	Person associated with
Black Revolution	Petroleum Production	–
Blue Revolution	Fish Production	Dr Arun Krishnan
Brown Revolution	Cocoa/Leather/ Non-Conventional Products	–
Grey Revolution	Fertilizers	–
Golden Revolution	Horticulture/ Honey/Fruit	Nirpakh Tutej
Golden Fiber Revolution	Jute Production	–
Pink Revolution	Onion and Prawn Production/ Pharmaceuticals	Durgesh Patel
Red Revolution	Meat and Tomato Production	Vishal Tewari
Silver Revolution	Egg/Poultry Production	Indira Gandhi
Silver Fiber Revolution	Cotton	–
Round Revolution	Potato	–
White Revolution (Or Operation Flood)	Dairy and Milk Production	Verghese Kurien
Green Revolution	Food Grains	Norman Borlaug, M.S Swaminathan, William Gaud (UK)
Yellow Revolution	Oil Seed Revolution (Especially Mustard and Sunflower)	Sam Pitroda
Protein Revolution	Higher Production (Technology driven 2nd Green Revolution)	PM Modi and Arun Jaitley

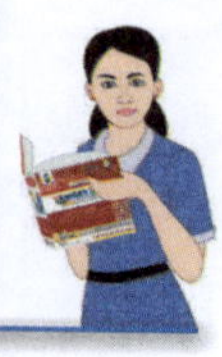

INTERNATIONAL ORGANIZATIONS, HEADQUARTERS AND HEAD

Organization name	Headquarters	Head
World Bank	Washington DC, US	David Malpass
International Monetary Fund (IMF)	Washington DC, US	Kristalina Georgieva
United Nations Children's Emergency Fund (UNICEF)	New York, US	Henrietta H Fore
United Nations Organization (UN)	New York, US	Antonio Guterres
United Nations General Assembly (UNGA)	New York, US	Abdulla Shahid
United Nations Population Fund (UNFPA)	New York, US	Dr Natalia Kanem
World Health Organization (WHO)	Geneva, Switzerland	Dr Tedros Adhanom Ghebreyesus
World Economic Forum (WEF)	Geneva, Switzerland	Klaus Schwab
International Labor Organization (ILO)	Geneva, Switzerland	Guy Ryder
World Trade Organization (WTO)	Geneva, Switzerland	Ngozi Okonjo-Iweala
World Intellectual Property Organization (WIPO)	Geneva, Switzerland	Daren Tang
World Meteorological Organization (WMO)	Geneva, Switzerland	David Grimes
United Nations Education Scientific and Cultural Organization (UNESCO)	Paris, France	Audrey Azoulay
International Atomic Energy Agency (IAEA)	Vienna, Austria	Rafael Mariano Grossi
International Maritime Organization (IMO)	London, UK	Kitack Lim
Commonwealth of Nations	London, UK	Queen Elizabeth II
Association of South East Nations (ASEAN)	Jakarta, Indonesia	Lim Jock Hoi

Contd...

Organization name	Headquarters	Head
North Atlantic Treaty Organization (NATO)	Brussels, Belgium	Jens Stoltenberg
International Cricket Council (ICC)	Dubai, UAE	Greg Barclay
Food and Agricultural Organization (FAO)	Rome, Italy	Qu Dongyu
International Court of Justice	Hague, Netherlands	Joan E. Donoghue
The Federation International de Football Association (FIFA)	Zurich, Switzerland	Gianni Infantino
United Nations Office on Drugs and Crime (UNODC)	Vienna, Austria	Ghada Fathi Waly
United Nations World Food Program (WFP)	Rome, Italy	David Beasley

PUBLIC SECTOR COMPANIES AND HEADQUARTERS

Company name	Establishment	Location
Airports Authority of India	1995	New Delhi
Bharat Electronics Limited (BEL)	1954	Bengaluru
Bharat Heavy Electricals Limited (BHEL)	1964	New Delhi
Bharat Petroleum Corporation Limited (BPCL)	1952	Mumbai
Bharat Sanchar Nigam Limited (BSNL)	2000	New Delhi
Coal India Limited (CIL)	1975	Kolkata
Container Corporation of India Ltd. (CONCOR)	1989	New Delhi
Engineers India Limited (EIL)	1965	New Delhi
Gas (India) Limited (GAIL)	1984	New Delhi
Hindustan Aeronautics Limited (HAL)	1940	Bengaluru
Hindustan Petroleum Corporation Limited (HPCL)	1974	Mumbai
Indian Oil Corporation Limited (IOCL)	1959	New Delhi
Mahanagar Telephone Nigam Limited (MTNL)	1986	New Delhi
National Aluminium Company Limited (NALCO)	1981	Bhubaneswar

Contd...

Company name	Establishment	Location
National Buildings Construction Corporation Limited (NBCC)	1960	New Delhi
National Mineral Development Corporation (NMDC) Limited	1958	Hyderabad
NLC India Limited	1956	Tamil Nadu
NTPC Limited	1975	New Delhi
Oil and Natural Gas Corporation Limited (ONGC)	1956	New Delhi
Oil India Limited (OIL)	1959	Assam
Power Finance Corporation Ltd.	1986	New Delhi
Power Grid Corporation of India Limited (PGCIL)	1989	Gurugram, Haryana
Rashtriya Ispat Nigam Ltd.	1982	Visakhapatnam
Rural Electrification Corporation Limited (REC)	1969	New Delhi
Shipping Corporation of India (SCI)	1961	Mumbai
Steel Authority of India (SAIL)	1954	New Delhi

LIST OF RESEARCH AND EDUCATIONAL INSTITUTES IN INDIA

Institute name	Location
Indian Agricultural Research Institute	New Delhi
Central Sugarcane Research Institute	Coimbatore
Central Forest Research Institute, Dehradun	Uttarakhand
Indian Cancer Research Institute	Mumbai
Indian Institute of Petroleum, Dehradun	Uttarakhand
Indian Meteorological Observatory	New Delhi
Indian Veterinary Research Institute, Bareilly	Uttar Pradesh
Central Rice Research Institute, Cuttack	Odisha
Central Potato Research Institute, Shimla	Himachal Pradesh
Central Fuel Research Institute, Dhanbad	Jharkhand
National Sugar Research Institute, Kanpur	Uttar Pradesh
Central Road Research Institute	New Delhi
Central Leather Research Institute, Chennai	Tamil Nadu
Central Drug Research Institute, Lucknow	Uttar Pradesh
National Institute of Virology, Pune	Maharashtra
Central Building Research Institute, Roorkee	Uttarakhand
Central Mining Research Institute, Dhanbad	Jharkhand
Central Electrochemical Research Institute, Karaikudi	Tamil Nadu
Central Coconut Research Institute, Chowki	Kerala
National Institute of Nutrition, Hyderabad	Telangana

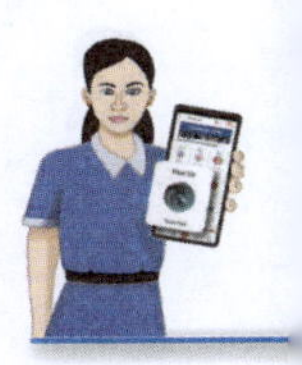

Contd...

Institute name	Location
National Tuberculosis Institute, Bengaluru	Karnataka
National Dairy Research Institute, Karnal	Haryana
National Botanical Research Institute, Lucknow	Uttar Pradesh
Archaeological Survey of India	New Delhi
Textile Research Institute, Ahmedabad	Gujarat
All India Malaria Research Institute	New Delhi
Central Leprosy Training and Research Institute	Tamil Nadu
National Institute of Oceanography	Goa
Central Glass and Ceramic Research Institute	West Bengal
Central Scientific Instruments Organization	Punjab
National Geophysical Research Institute Hyderabad	Telangana
National Aeronautical Laboratory, Bengaluru	Karnataka
Vallabhbhai Patel Chest Institute	New Delhi
High Altitude Research Laboratory	Jammu and Kashmir
Central Marine Research Station	Tamil Nadu
Council of Scientific and Industrial Research	New Delhi
Indian Space Research Organization (ISRO)	Bengaluru, Karnataka
Indira Gandhi Center for Atomic Research	Tamil Nadu
Institute of Plasma Research	Gujarat

Institute name	Location
National Botanical Research Institute	Uttar Pradesh
National Council for Cement and Building Materials, Hyderabad	Telangana
National Metallurgical Laboratory	Jharkhand
National Tuberculosis Institute	Karnataka
Seismic Research Center	Karnataka
Wool Research Association	Maharashtra
Structural Engineering Research Center	Tamil Nadu
National Institute of Occupational Health	Gujarat
National Environmental Engineering Research Institute	Maharashtra
National Institute of Communicable Diseases	New Delhi
Uranium Corporation of India	Jharkhand
Radio Astronomy Center	Tamil Nadu
Electronics Corporation of India	Telangana
Bhabha Atomic Research Center	Mumbai
Tata Institute of Fundamental Research	Maharashtra
Vikram Sarabhai Space Center	Kerala
Indian Scientific Satellite Project	Karnataka
Space Application Center	Gujarat
Center of Earth Science Studies	Kerala
Nuclear Fuel Complex	Telangana

Contd...

PURPOSES OF IMAGE OR MAP

- Aids in learning the position of states and their shared boundaries with other states and countries.
- Apart from that, the date of establishment of all states is also given.

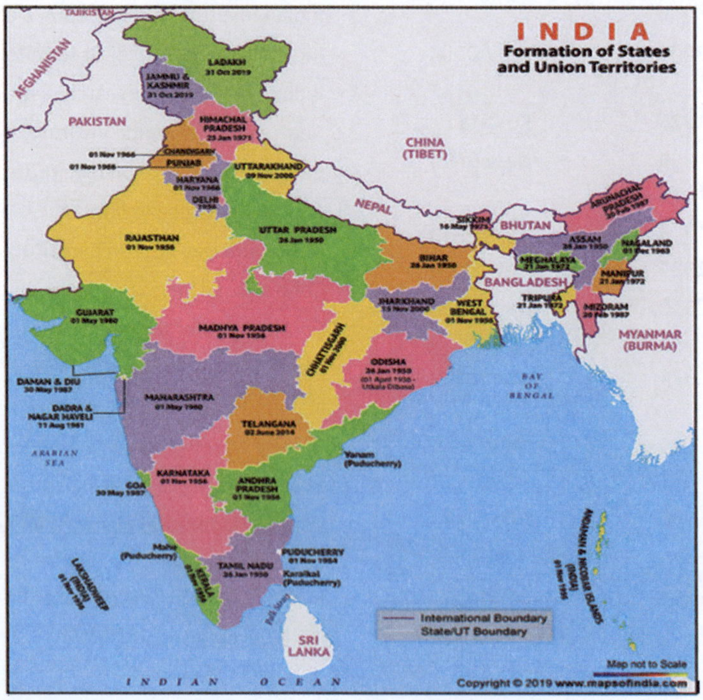

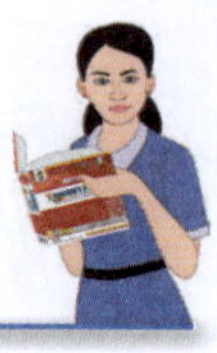

- Special focus should be on Jammu and Kashmir, Ladakh as both are declared two new Union territories on 144th Birth anniversary of Sardar Vallabhbhai Patel, i.e., 31st October, 2019. Radha Krishna Mathur has been appointed as the first Lieutenant-Governor (L-G) of Ladakh and Girish Chandra Murmu, that of Jammu and Kashmir (J&K).

INDIAN STATES—THEIR CAPITALS, IMPORTANT FESTIVALS AND DANCE FORMS

State	Capital	Festival	Dance forms	Monuments
Andhra Pradesh	Amaravati	Sankranti, Deepothsavam Tyagaraja Festival, Ugadi (New year), Rottela Panduga Brahmotsavam	Kuchipudi, Burrakatha, Veeranatyam, Butta Bommalu, Tappeta Gullu, Dhimsa, Kolattam, Vilasini Natyam	Tirupati Balaji Temple
Arunachal Pradesh	Itanagar	Losar Festival	Aji Lamu, Roppi, Lion and peacock dance, Chalo, Popir, Bardo Chham, Ponung	
Assam	Dispur	Bihu, Porag, Gaan-Ngai, Majuli festival, Dehing Patkai Festival, Ambubachi festival	Sattriya, Bihu, Bagurumba, Ali Ai Ligang, Ojapali, Bohuwa, Bhortal, Jhumur	
Bihar	Patna	Chhath, Rajgir Dance festival, Jivitputrika, Bihula, Madhushravani	Kajari Dance, Jumari, Bidesia, Jat-Jatin, Jhijhya, Fagua, Domkach, Sohar Khilona	Golghar, Pathar ki Masjid, Sher Shah's Tomb, Vishnupad Temple
Chhattisgarh	Raipur	Bastar Dussehra	Pandwani, Raut Nacha, Gendi dance, Panthi, Karma, Sua Nacha, Saila dance	Bastar Fort
Delhi	Delhi	Bharat Rang Mahotsav, Qutub Festival, Sabrang Utsav, Jahan-e- Khusrau		Feroz Shah Kotla, Humayun Tomb, Jama Masjid, Jantar-Mantar, Lakshmi Narayan Temple, Moti Masjid, President House, Purana Qila, Qutub Minar, Red Fort, Safdarjung Tomb
Goa	Panaji	Feast of Three Kings, Sunburn Festival, Gokulastami, Feast of St Francis Xavier, Mando Festival	Talgadi, Mando, Suvari, Dasarawadan, Kunbi dance, Fugadi, Dhalo, Ghode Modni, Goff, Dekhni dance, Dhangar, Tonyamel	
Gujarat	Gandhinagar	Navaratri, Kite Festival, Saptak Music Festival, Holi	Garba, Dandiya Raas, Garbi, Tippani, Bhavai, Vinchhudo, Hudo, kahalya	Sabarmati Ashram, Somnath Temple, Bhuj Fort
Haryana	Chandigarh	Surajkund Craft Mela, Baisakhi Festival	Gugga Dance, Khoria dance, Rasleela, Dhamal, Phag, loor , Daph dance	
Himachal Pradesh	Shimla	Minjar Mela, Kullu Dussehra, Jwalamukhi Fair, Losar Festival	Kullu Nati, Namgen, Chham dance, Thoda, Dandras, Ghuregi, Jhora, Dangi	
Jammu and Kashmir	Srinagar	Accession Day, Sont, Galdan Namchot, Jeth Ashtami, Mela at Hemis Gompa, Har Navami, Chhari Festival, Tulip Festival	Dumhal, Kud dance, Bhand Jashan, Bhand Pather, Bacha Nagma, Hafiza, Wuegi-Nachun, Hikat, Rauf	Charar-E-Sharif, Nishant Garden, Shalimar Garden
Jharkhand	Ranchi	Tusu festival	Chhau Dance, Jhumair, Phagua, Karma	

Contd...

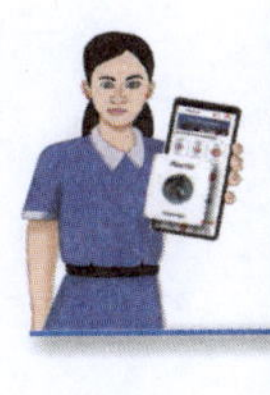

State	Capital	Festival	Dance forms	Monuments
Karnataka	Bengaluru	Makar Sankranti, Ugadi, Japan Habba, Karaga, Kanakadasa Jayanthi, Ugadi, Ganesha Chaturthi		Hampi, Mysore Palace, Gol Gumbaz
Kerala	Thiruvananthapuram	Onam, Theyyam, Poorum, Nehru Trophy Boat Race	Kathakali, Mohiniattam, Kaikottikali, Thumbithullal, Ottamthullal, Koodiyattam, Chakyar Koothu, Theyyam, Kolkali, Thiruvathirakali, Theyyam	
Ladakh (UT)	Leh	Sindhu Darshan Festival, Hemis Festival		
Madhya Pradesh	Bhopal	Khajuraho Dance Festival, Malwa Utsav, Tansen Music Festival, Mandu Festival	Matki, Gangaur, Badhai, Baredi, Naurata, Ahirai, Bhagoria, Karma dance, Gaur maria dance, Kaksar dance	Khajuraho temples, Sanchi stupas, Datia fort
Maharashtra	Mumbai	GudiPadva, Rishi Panchami, Ganesh Chaturdi, Kala Ghoda Arts Festival	Pavri Nach, Lavani, Dhangari Gaja, Dindi and kala, Tamasha	Ajanta- Ellora caves, Bibi ka Maqbara, Elephanta cave, Gateway of India, Kanheri Fort
Manipur	Imphal	Kut festival, Orange festival, Sangai Festival	Manipuri dance or Jagoi, Khamba Thoibi dance, Pung Cholom, Thang ta, Dhol Cholom, Lai Haraoba	Shri Govindajee Temple, Kangla Fort
Meghalaya	Shillong	Cherry Blossom Festival	Nongkrem, Ka Shad Suk Mynsiem	
Mizoram	Aizawl	Chapchar Kut Festival, Zo Festival	Khuallam, Cheraw (Bamboo dance), Sarlamkai/Solakai	
Nagaland	Kohima	Metemneo Festival, Hornbill Festival	Changlo-Sua-lua	
Odisha	Bhubaneswar	Jagannath Ratha Yatra	Odissi, Ghumura dance, Ruk Mar Nacha, GotiPua, Chhou, Chaiti ghoda, Danda Nata, Changu	Jagannath Temple, Sun Temple, Konark Sun Temple
Punjab	Chandigarh	Teej, Tikka, Holla Mohalla, Lohri, Gurupurab, Baisakhi	Bhangra, Gidda, Jhumar, Luddi, Dankara	Golden Temple
Rajasthan	Jaipur	Camel Festival, Teej, Pushkar Fair, Baneshwar fair, Gangaru, Chaksu fair, Urs at Ajmer, Desert festival, Mewar Festival, Gangaur Festival, Kolayat Fair	Ghoomar, Kalbelia, Bhavai, Sapera dance, Kachchhi Ghodi, Kathputli, Bhopa, Chang, Terahtaali, Gair dance, Tejaji	Adhai din ka Jhonpra, Bharatpur Fort, Ajmer Sharif Dargah, Dilwara Jain Temple, Hawa Mahal, Jaigarh fort, Jodhpur fort, Nahargarh fort, Vijaya Stambha
Sikkim	Gangtok	International Flower festival, Saga Dawa	Singhi Chham, Khukuri Naach, Chu Faat, Yak Chham, Tashi Yangku, Maruni	
Tamil Nadu	Chennai	Pongal, Deepavali, Panguni Uthiram, Puthandu (Tamil new year), Thaipoosam, Jangura Habba, Vaikunda Ekadasi	Bharatanatyam, Mayilattam, Bommalattam, Kummi, Kai Silambattam, Karagattam, Kolattam, Kavadi	Meenakshi Amman temple, Saint George fort
Tripura	Agartala	Karachi Puja, Tripureshwari temple Festival, Hornbill Festival, Lai Haraoba	Garia Dance, Hozagiri dance, Bizu, Lebang Boomani, Hai-Hak, Jhum, Sangrai- Mog	Mata Tripura Sundari temple, Unakoti

Contd...

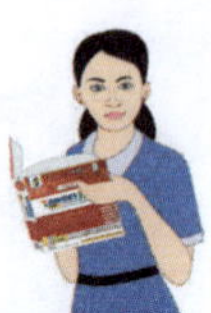

State	Capital	Festival	Dance forms	Monuments
Uttar Pradesh	Lucknow	Brahmotsav, Ram Navami, Ban Yatra, Sravana Festival, Kans Ka Mela, Taj Mahotsav, Kumbh Mela	Kathak, Chholia, Raslila, Khyal, Nautanki, Ramlila, Naqal, Svanga, Charkula dance	Fatehpur Sikri, Agra Fort, Sarnath Buddhist ruins, Aram bagh, Bada Imambara, Chhota Imambara, Deewan-e-Khas, Tomb of Itmad-ud-Daula, Taj Mahal, Shish Mahal
West Bengal	Kolkata	Dussehra, Gangasagar Mela, Poush Mela, Ramakrishna Utsav, Vasant Panchami, Naba Barsha, Nandikar National Theater festival, Kobita Utsav (Poetry festival)	Chhau, Gambhira, Kalikapatadi, Domni, Kathi	Shantiniketan, Belur Math, Victoria Memorial

LIST OF HILL RANGES IN INDIA AND THEIR LOCATIONS

Hill Ranges

Hill Range	States
Aravallis	Gujarat, Rajasthan, Haryana
Anamalai Hills	Kerala and Tamil Nadu
Cardamom Hills	Kerala and Tamil Nadu
Eastern Ghats	Tamil Nadu, Karnataka, Andhra Pradesh, Odisha, West Bengal
Garo, Khasi, Jaintia Hills	Meghalaya
Karakoram	Ladakh in Jammu and Kashmir
Nallamala Hills	Andhra Pradesh
Nilgiri Hills	Tamil Nadu, Kerala and Karnataka
Palani Hills	Tamil Nadu
Pir Panjal	Himachal Pradesh, Jammu and Kashmir
Vindhyas	Gujarat, Madhya Pradesh, Uttar Pradesh
Satpura	Gujarat, Maharashtra, Madhya Pradesh, Chhattisgarh
Seshachalam Hills	Andhra Pradesh
Western Ghats	Tamil Nadu, Kerala, Karnataka, Goa, Maharashtra

Highest Peak

Highest Peak in India is Kanchenjunga (8586 m) located in Sikkim. Kanchenjunga is the **third highest Mountain** in the world. First two highest mountains in the world are:

1. Mount Everest: 8,848.86 mts
2. K2 also known as Godwin Austin: 8,611 mts
3. Kanchenjunga: 8,586 mts

IMPORTANT PASSES

Name of the Pass	Location	Connects
Shipki La	Himachal Pradesh	Shimla with Tibet
Nathula	Sikkim	Sikkim and Tibet
Rohtang Pass	Himachal Pradesh	Manali and Lahul
Bhor Ghat	Maharashtra	Mumbai and Pune
Thal Ghat	Maharashtra	Nasik and Mumbai
Pal Ghat	Tamil Nadu	Kerala with Tamil Nadu

SUPERLATIVES IN INDIA

Question	Answer
Largest Lake	Wular (Kashmir)
Largest Delta	Sunderban Delta
Largest Cave Temple	Ellora (Maharashtra)
Largest State in Population	Uttar Pradesh
Largest Dome	Gol Gumbaz, Bijapur
Largest Mosque	Jama Masjid, Delhi
Highest Peak	Nanda Devi
Highest Rainfall	Mawsynram (Meghalaya)
Highest Dam	Bhakra Nangal Dam, Punjab
Highest Gateway	Buland Darwaza, Fatehpur Sikri
Highest Tower	Qutub Minar
Highest Waterfalls	Jog Falls (Karnataka)
Highest Civilian Award	Bharat Ratna
Highest Award for gallantry	Param Vir Chakra
Largest Desert	Thar (Rajasthan)
Longest Road	Grand Trunk Road
Largest Tunnel	Jawahar Tunnel (Banihal, Kashmir)
Longest Dam	Hirakud Dam (Orissa)

Contd...

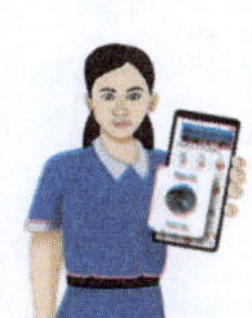

Question	Answer
Tallest Statue	Statue of Gomateshwara in Karnataka
Biggest Museum	Indian Museum, Calcutta
Longest River	The Ganges
Largest District	Ladakh (J&K)

NATIONAL SYMBOLS OF INDIA

Title	Symbol	Picture
National Animal	Tiger	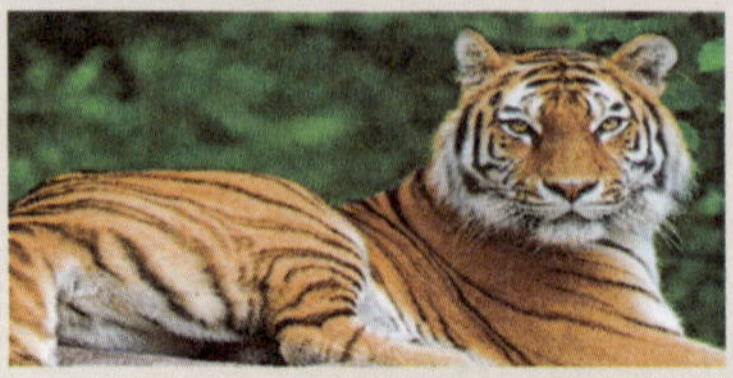
National Anthem	Jan Gana Mana	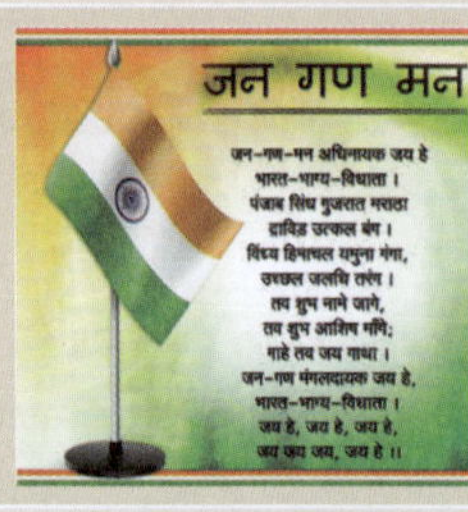
National Aquatic Animal	River Dolphin	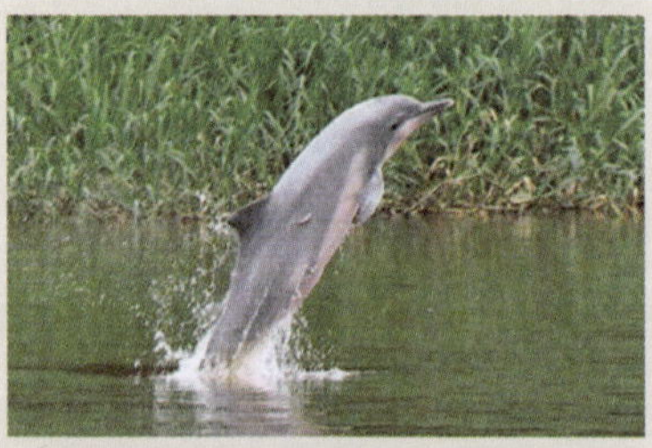
National Bird	Peacock	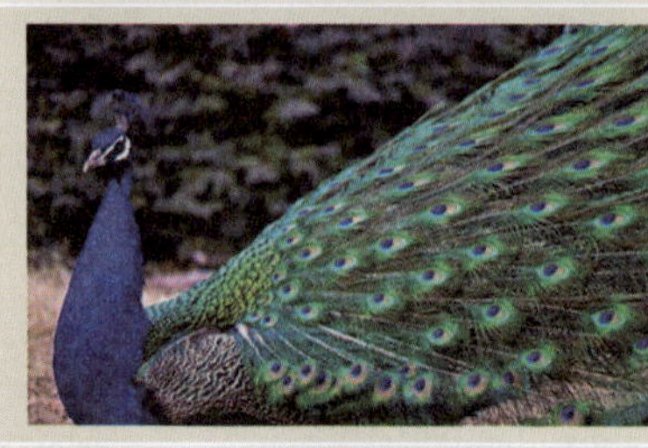
National Emblem	State Emblem of India	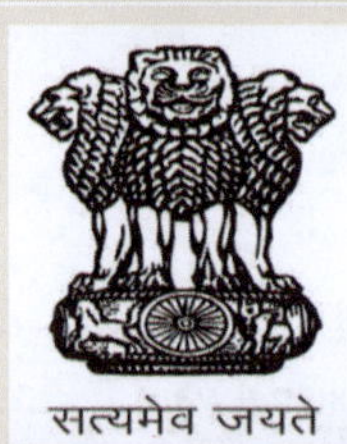
National Flag	Tiranga	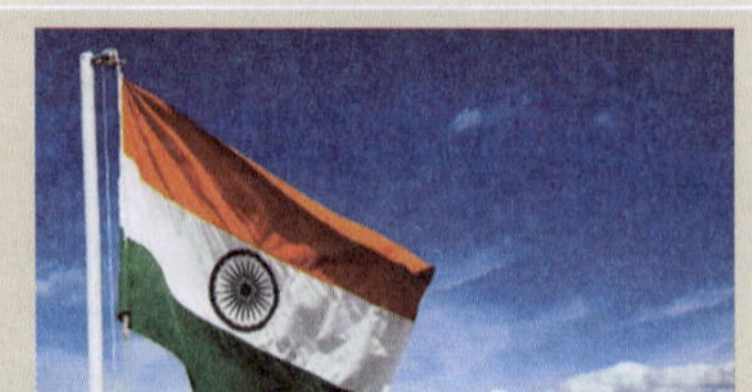

Contd...

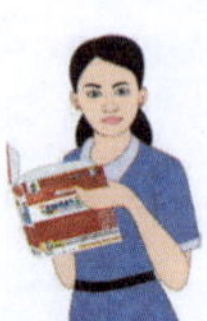

Title	Symbol	Picture
National Flower	Lotus	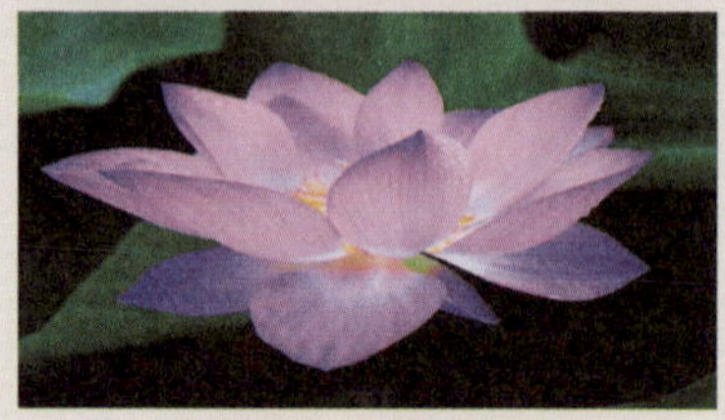
National Fruit	Mango	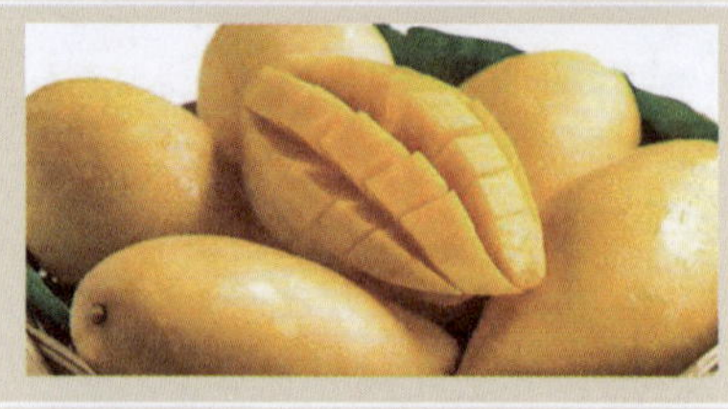
National River	Ganga	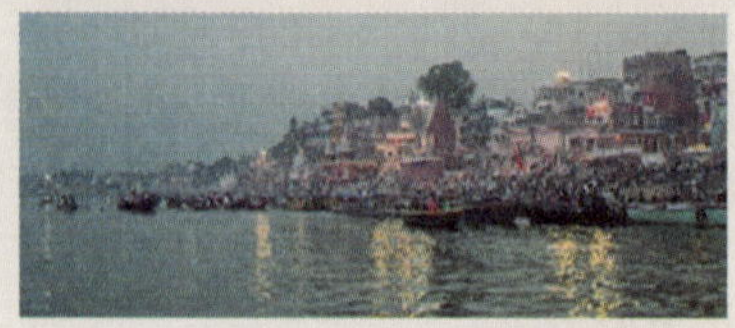
National Song	Vande Mataram	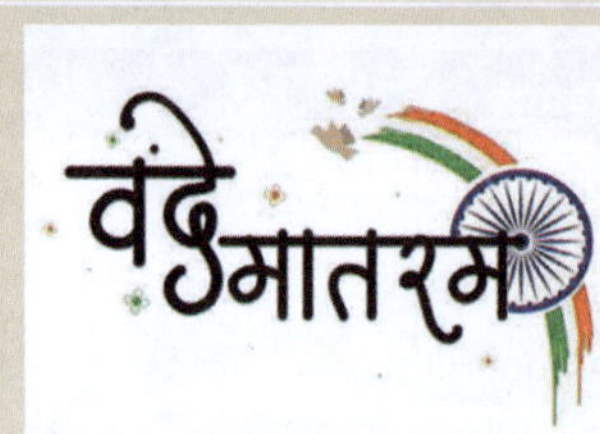

FAMOUS BOOKS AND AUTHORS FROM ANCIENT INDIA

Any civilized society cannot be imagined without books and authors. Educated people shape and mold the society and so we must know about the books which have been part of our life since ancient time.

Books	Authors
Abhigyan Shakuntalam	Kalidasa
Aihole Prasasti	Ravi Kriti
Amarakosha	Amarasimha
Arthashastra	Kautilya
Astadhyayi	Panini
Brihat Samhita	Varahamihira
Buddha Charita	Asvaghosa
Charaka Samhita	Charaka
Gatha Saptashati	Hala
Gita Govinda	Jayadev
Indica	Megasthanese
Kathasaritsagar	Somdeva
Kamasutra	Vatsayana
Mahabhasya	Patanjali
Mrichhakatika	Sudraka

Contd...

Books	Authors
Mudrarakshasa	Visakhdatta
Naishadhacharitra	Sri Harsha
Natyashastra	Bharata
Navratna	Virsena
Nitisara	Kamandaka
Panch tantra	Vishnu Sharma
Prashnottarmalika	Amoghavarsha
Raghuvansam	Kalidasa
Rajtarangini	Kalhana
Ratnavali	Harsha Vardhan

BOOKS AND AUTHORS

Authors	Books
K S Vijayanath	'Sabarimala Vijnaanakosham'
Alfredo Coveli	'Vahana Masterclass'
R. Giridharan	Right Under Our Nose
R. Kaushik	India's 71-Year Test: The Journey to Triumph in Australia
Lt. Gen. Konsam Himalay Singh	'Making of a General-A Himalayan Echo'
Romila Thapar	'Gazing Eastwards: Of Buddhist Monks and Revolutionaries in China, 1957'
S Y Quraishi	'The Population Myth: Islam, Family Planning and Politics in India'
Vidhu Vinod Chopra and Abhijat Joshi'	'Unscripted: Conversations on Life and Cinema'
Ramachandra Guha	'The Commonwealth of Cricket'
Waman Subha Prabhu	'Manohar Parrikar-Off the Record'
Dr APJM Nazema Maraikayar and Dr Y S Rajan	'Abdul Kalam- Ninaivugalukku Maranamillai'
Mohamed Zeeshan	Flying Blind: India's Quest for Global Leadership
Gautam Chikermane	'India 2030: The Rise of a Rajasic Nation'
Dr Abhishek Singhvi and Prof. Khagesh Gautam	'The Law of Emergency Powers: Comparative Common Law Perspectives'
Arun Sengupta and Partha Mukherjee	'Soumitra Chatterjee: A Life in Cinema, Theatre, Poetry and Painting"
Andre De Grasse and Robert Budd	'Race With Me!'
APJ Abdul Kalam	Wings of Fire
Khushwant Singh	Truth, Love and Little Malice
Milkha singh	The Race of My Life
L K Advani	My Country My Life

Contd...

Authors	Books
K Natwar singh	One Life is Not Enough
Yuvraj singh	The Test of My Life
Jawaharlal Nehru	An Autobiography
Sachin Tendulkar	Playing it My Way
IK Gujral	Matters of Discretion
Abhinav Bindra	A Shot at History
Kapil Dev	Straight from the Heart
JB Kripalani (Acharya Kripalani)	My Times
Subhash Chandra	The Z Factor
M K Gandhi	My Experiments with Truth
Richard Branson	Losing My virginity
Stephen Hawking	My Brief History
Michael Jackson	Moon Walk
Alice Schroeder	The Snowball: Warren Buffett and Business of Life
Pandit Ravi Shankar	Raga Mala
Zubin Mehta	The Score of My Life
Nelson Mandela	Long Walk to Freedom
Helen Keller	The Story of My Life
Shatrugan Sinha	Anything But Khamosh
Muhammad Ali	The Greatest: My Own Story
Prabhu Desai	The Nice Guy who Finished First (Rahul Dravid, Biography)
PT Usha (Athlete)	Golden Girl
Usain Bolt (Athlete)	Faster Than Lightening: My Autobiography
Kevin Pietersen (South African Cricketer)	KP: The Autobiography
David Beckham (Football player)	My World My Side
Albert Einstein	Autobiographical Notes
Bill Clinton	My Life
Hillary Clinton	Living History
Salim Ali (Ornithologist)	The Fall of a Sparrow
V R K Iyer	Wandering in Many Worlds
Phoolan Devi	The Bandit Queen of India
Dilip Kumar	The Substance and the Shadow
Leo Tolstoy	My Confession
Marlon Brando	Songs My Mother Taught
Maxim Gorky	My Childhood
Aero Smith	Walk this Way
Benazir Bhutto	Daughter of the Destiny
Wasim Akram (Pakistan Cricketer)	Wasim: Autobiography
Shoaib Akhtar (Pakistan Fast bowler)	Controversially Yours
Lance Armstrong	It's Not About the Bike: My Journey Back to Life

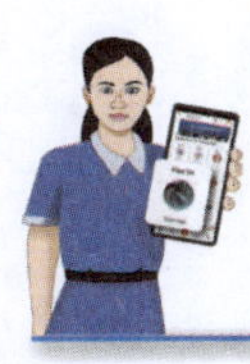

Contd...

Authors	Books
Nirad C Chaudhuri	The Autobiography of An Unknown Indian
Barack Obama	Dreams from My Father
R K Narayan	My Days
Amrita Pritam	Revenue Stamp: An Autobiography
Malala Yousafzai	I am Malala
Benjamin Franklin	The Autobiography of Benjamin Franklin
Mahatma Gandhi	Story of my Experiments with Truth
Agatha Christie	An Autobiography of Agatha Christie
Jawaharlal Nehru	An Autobiography
Sachin Tendulkar	Playing it My Way
Kapil Dev	Straight From the Heart
Hellen Keller	Story of My Life
Khushwant Singh	Truth Love and a Little Malice
Bhagat Singh	Why I am an Atheist
Babur	Baburnama
Malcolm X	The Autobiography of Malcolm X
Robert T Washington	Up from Slavery
Laura Hillenbrand	Unbroken

STATE WISE NATIONAL PARKS, TIGER RESERVES AND WILDLIFE SANCTUARIES

- National parks are the reserved areas of land owned by govt. which are highly restricted to preserve the overall flora, fauna, landscapes and historical objects. There are total **106 national parks in India**. **First national park** established was **Hailey National Park** in 1936, now known as **Jim Corbett National Park**. Largest national park is Hemis National Park situated in Ladakh and smallest national park is South Button Island National Park situated in Andaman and Nicobar Islands.
- A tiger reserve is a habitat majorly owned by tigers, so managed as an inviolate area. There are total **53 tiger reserves in India**. **First tiger reserve** established was **Jim Corbett** established in 1936. Largest tiger reserve is Nagarjunsagar-Srisailam, situated in Andhra Pradesh and smallest tiger reserve is Bor tiger reserve, situated in Maharashtra.
- A wildlife sanctuary is an area owned by govt. or pvt. agency for the protection of particular species of flora or fauna from poaching, hunting, predation. Here, restrictions are comparatively less and is open for public visits. There are total 567 wildlife sanctuaries in India. First wildlife sanctuary established in India is Senchal Wildlife Sanctuary in 1915 located at Darjeeling District of West Bengal. Largest wildlife sanctuary in India is Indian Wild Ass Sanctuary in Gujarat and the smallest wildlife sanctuary is Mayureswar Wildlife Sanctuary in Maharashtra.

State/UT	National Parks	Tiger Reserves	Wildlife Sanctuaries
Andaman and Nicobar Islands	• Galathea National Park • Mahatma Gandhi Marine (Wandoor) National Park • Campbell Bay National Park • Mount Harriet National Park • Rani Jhansi Marine National Park • Saddle peak National Park • Middle Button Island National Park • North Button Island • National Park • South Button Island National Park		• Bamboo Island WLS • Barren Island WLS • Chanel Island WLS • Peacock Island WLS • Turtle Islands WLS
Andhra Pradesh	• Papikonda National Park • Sri Venkateswara National Park • Rajiv Gandhi (Rameswaram) National Park	Nagarjunasagar Srisailam	• Kolleru Bird Sanctuary • Nelapattu Bird Sanctuary • Pulicat Lake Bird Sanctuary • Coringa Wildlife Sanctuary • Nagarjunsagar-Srisailam Tiger Reserve • Sri Venkateswara National Park • Rollapadu Wildlife Sanctuary • Sri Lankamalleswara Wildlife Sanctuary • Krishna Wildlife Sanctuary • Kaundinya Wildlife Sanctuary • Gundla Brahmeswaram Wildlife Sanctuary • Sri Penusila Narasimha Wildlife Sanctuary • Kambalakonda Wildlife Sanctuary

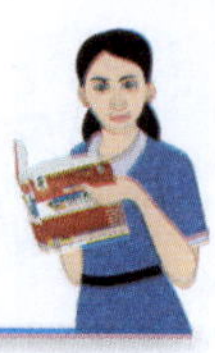

Contd...

State/UT	National Parks	Tiger Reserves	Wildlife Sanctuaries
Arunachal Pradesh	• Mouling National Park • Namdapha National Park	• Namdapha • Kamlang Tiger Reserve • Pakke Tiger Reserve	
Assam	• Nameri National Park • Manas National Park • Dibru- Saikhowa National Park • Kaziranga National Park • Orang National Park • Dehing Patkai National Park • Raimona National Park	• Manas • Nameri • Orang Tiger Reserve Kaziranga	
Bihar	• Valmiki National Park • Vikramshila Gangetic Dolphin Sanctuary • Kanwar Lake Bird Sanctuary	Valmiki	• Gautam Buddha WLS • Valmiki WLS • Kaimur WLS • Udaypur WLS • Pant (Rajgir) WLS • Kusheshwar Asthan Bird WLS
Chhattisgarh	• Indravati National Park • Kanger Valley National Park • Guru Ghasidas (Sanjay) National Park	• Udanti- Sitanadi • Achanakmar • Indravati • Guru Ghasidas	
Goa	Bhagwan Mahavir (Mollem) National Park		• Cotigao Wildlife Sanctuary • Netravali Wildlife Sanctuary • Mhadei Wildlife Sanctuary • Salim Ali Bird Sanctuary • Bondla Wildlife Sanctuary • Bhagwan Mahavir Sanctuary
Gujarat	• Gir National Park • Blackbuck National Park • Gulf of Kutch National Park • Vansda National Park • Marine National Park		• Gaga Great Indian Bustard WLS • Gir WLS • Girnar WLS • Lala Great Indian Bustard WLS • Marine (Gulf of Kutch) WLS • Nal Sarovar Bird Santuary • Narayan Sarovar (chinkara) WLS • Porbandar Lake WLS • Thol Lake WLS • Wild Ass WLS • Kacchh Desert WLS • Ratanmahal Sloth Bear WLS • Ramparavidi WLS • Khijadiya Bird WLS • Barda WLS • Shoolpaneshwar WLS • Balaram-Ambaji WLS
Haryana	• Sultanpur National Park • Kalesar National Park		• Bhindawas Wildlife Sanctuary • Sultanpur Bird Sanctuary
Himachal Pradesh	• Pin Valley National Pak • Simbalbara National Park • Inderkilla National Park • Khirganga National Park • Great Himalayan National Park		• Kalatop- Khajjiar WLS • Tunda WLS • Shimla Water Catchment WLS • Dhauladar WLS • Rakchham Chitkul (Sangla Valley) WLS • Pong Dam Lake WLS • Renuka WLS • Shikari Devi WLS • Chandratal WLS • Sechu Tuan Nala Wildlife Sanctuary • Tundah Wildlife Sanctuary • Kugti Wildlife Sanctuary • Nargu Wildlife Sanctuary

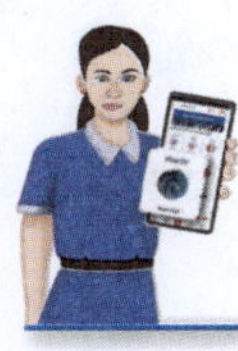

Contd...

State/UT	National Parks	Tiger Reserves	Wildlife Sanctuaries
Jammu and Kashmir	• Dachigam National Park • Salim Ali National Park • Kishtwar National Park • Kazinag National Park		• Karakoram WLS • Gulmarg WLS • Hirapora WLS • Trikuta WLS • Ramnagar Rakha WLS • Kanji WLS • Changtang WLS
Ladakh	Hemis National Park		
Jharkhand	• Betla National Park • Hazaribagh National Park	Palamau	• Dalma Wildlife Sanctuary • Lawalong WLS • Parasnath WLS • Palkot WLS
Karnataka	• Bandipur National Park • Anshi National Park • Bannerghata National Park • Kudremukh National Park • Nagarhole (Rajiv Gandhi) National Park	• Bandipur • Bhadra • Dandeli – Anshi • Nagarhole • Kudremukha • Biligiriranga Hills	• Someshwara WLS • Bhadra WLS • Bhimgad WLS • Brahmagiri WLS • Cauvery WLS • Pushpagiri WLS • Sharavathi Valley WLS
Kerala	• Eravikulam National Park • Mathikettan Shola National Park • Periyar National Park • Silent Valley National Park • Anamudi Shola National Park • Pambadum Shola National Park	• Periyar • Parambikulam	• Periyar Wildlife Sanctuary • Chinnar Wildlife Sanctuary • Aralam WLS • Chimmony WLS • Idukki WLS • Malabar WLS
Madhya Pradesh	• Pench (Indira Priyadarshini) National Park Bandhavgarh National Park • Kanha National Park • Panna National Park • Sanjay National Park • Satpura National Park • Madhav National Park • Van Vihar National Park • Mandla Plant Fossils National Park	• Kanha • Pench • Bandhavgarh • Panna • Bori-Satpura • Sanjay Dubri • Ratapani	• Gandhi Sagar WLS • National Chambal WLS • Pachmarhi WLS • Kuno WLS • Panna WLS • Pench WLS • Veerangna Durgawati WLS • Bori WLS • Sanjay Dubri WLS • Narsinghgarh WLS
Maharashtra	• Navegaon National Park • Sanjay Gandhi (Borivali) • National Park Chandoli National Park • Gugamal National Park • Tadoba National Park	• Melghat • Tadoba- Andhari • Sahyadri • Bor • Navegaon- Nazgira	• Koyana WLS • Painganga WLS • Bhimashankar WLS • Tungareshwar WLS • Great Indian Bustard WLS
Manipur	• Sirohi National Park • Keibul Lamjao National Park		Yangoupokpi-Lokchao WLS
Meghalaya	• Nokrek National Park • Balphakram National Park		
Mizoram	• Murlen National Park • Phawngpui Blue Mountain National Park	Dampa	• Dampa WLS (TR) • Ngengpui WLS • Baghmara Pitcher Plant WLS
Nagaland	Ntangki National Park		• Fakim WLS • Rangapahar WLS
Odisha	• Simlipal National Park • Bhitarkanika National Park • Nandankanan National Park	• Similipal • Satkosia • Sunabeda	• Baisipalli WLS • Chilika (Nalaban) WLS • Hadgarh WLS • Satkosia Gorge WLS

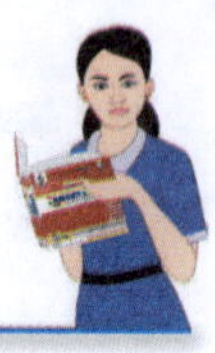

Contd...

State/UT	National Parks	Tiger Reserves	Wildlife Sanctuaries
Punjab	• Abohar National Park • Harike Wetland • Jhajjar Bachauli National Park • Bir Moti bagh National Park • Bir Bhadson National Park • Mahendra Zoological Park (Chatt Bir zoo)		• Abohar WLS • Harike Lake WLS • Nangal WLS • Jhajjar Bacholi WLS
Rajasthan	• Sariska Tiger Reserve • Ranthambore National Park • MukundraHils (Darrah) National Park • Keoladeo Ghana National Park • Desert National Park • Mount Abu Wildlife Sanctuary	• Ranthambore • Sariska • Mukandra Hills • Darrah • Ramgarh Vishdhari	• Kailadevi WLS • Mount Abu WLS • Sariska WLS • Sawai Man Singh WLS • Bandh Baratha WLS • Jawahar Sagar WLS • Darrah WLS • Keladevi WLS • Ramgarh Vishdhari WLS
Sikkim	Khangchendzonga National Park		• Fambong Lho WLS • Kitam WLS (Bird) • Maenam WLS
Tamil Nadu	• Mudumalai National Park • Mukurthi National Park • Indira Gandhi (Anamalai) National Park • Guindy National Park • Gulf of Mannar • Marine National Park • Palani Hills National Park	• Kalakad- Mundanthurai • Anamalai • Mudumalai • Sathyamangalam • Meghamalai	• Indira Gandhi (Anamalai) WLS • Karaivetti WLS • Pulicat Lake WLS • Vedanthangal WLS • Kalakad WLS
Telangana	• Mahavir Harina Vanasthali National Park • Kasu Brahmananda Reddy National Park Mrugavani National Park	• Nagarjunasagar Srisailam Kawal • Amrabad	
Tripura	• Clouded Leopard National Park • Bison (Rajbari) National Park		• Gumti WLS • Rowa WLS • Trishna WLS
Uttar Pradesh	Dudhwa National Park	• Dudhwa • Philibhit • Amangarh (Buffer of Corbett Tiger Reserve) • Katerniaghat	• Bakhira WLS • Chandraprabha WLS • Dr Bhimarao Ambedkar Bird Sanctuary • Hastinapur WLS • Kaimur WLS • Turtle WLS • Pilibhit WLS • Jai Prakash Narayan Bird WLS • Kishanpur WLS • Okhala Bird Sanctuary • Patna WLS • Nawabganj Bird WLS • Saman Bird Sanctuary • Sur Sarovar Bird WLS • Vijay Sagar WLS • Katarniaghat • Ranipur
Uttarakhand	• Corbett • Rajaji	• Corbett • Rajaji	• Askot Musk Deer WLS • Nandhaur WLS • Binsar WLS • Kedarnath WLS • Mussoorie WLS • Govind Pashu Vihar WLS • Sonanadi WLS

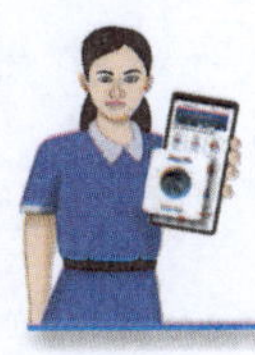

Contd...

State/UT	National Parks	Tiger Reserves	Wildlife Sanctuaries
West Bengal	• Buxa National Park • Neora Valley National Park • Gorumara National Park • Singalila National Park • Jaldapara National Park • Sunderbans National Park	• Sunderbans • Buxa	• Sunderbans Wildlife Sanctuary • Chintamani Kar Bird Sanctuary • Haliday Island WLS • Ballavpur WLS • Lothian Island WLS • Mahananda WLS

CENSUS IN INDIA

Census is the process of collecting and analyzing the statistical data regarding the population of a country.

Census operation was started during the period of Maurya dynasty. It has been conducted uninterruptedly from the year 1881. Census 2011 was the 15th census of India and 7th census after independence of India. This was conducted in two segments:

1. Population enumeration
2. Housing and house listing

Census 2011 Report

- Motto: Our Census, Our Future

Population	Total	1,210,854,977
	Males	623,724,568
	Females	587,469,294
Literacy	Total	74%
	Males	82.10%
	Females	65.46%
Density of population	Per sq. km	382
Sex ratio	Per 1000 males	940 females
Child sex ratio (up to 6 years)	Per 1000 males	914 females

- The Census of 2011 was released on 31st March 2011 by Union Home Secretary and RGI of India.
- The overall increase in population during 2001- 2011 is 181 million.

Feature	State
Highest populated state Least populous state	Uttar Pradesh Sikkim
Highest populated UT Least populous UT	Delhi Lakshadweep
Most Populated City Least Populated City	Mumbai (Maharashtra) Kapurthala (Punjab)
Most Populated District Least Populated District	Thane (Maharashtra) Dibang Valley (Arunachal Pradesh)
Highest and Lowest urban population in India (state and UT)	Maharashtra Lakshadweep
Highest and Lowest rural population in India (state and UT)	Uttar Pradesh Lakshadweep
Highest sex ratio in state Highest sex ratio in UT	Kerala Pondicherry
Lowest sex ratio in state Lowest sex ratio in UT	Mahe, Pondicherry Daman, Daman and Diu
Highest child sex ratio in state Lowest child sex ratio in state	Kerala Haryana
Highest Literacy Rate in State Highest Literacy Rate in UT	Kerala Lakshadweep

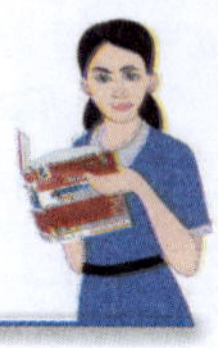

Contd...

Feature	State
Lowest Literacy Rate in State Lowest Literacy Rate in UT	Bihar Dadra and Nagar Haveli
Highest Literacy Rate District Lowest Literacy Rate District	Serchhipp (Mizoram) 98.28% Alirajpur (Madhya pradesh) 36.10%
Highest Density State High Density UT	West Bengal (88,752 sq.km) Delhi (11,297 per sq.km)

IMPORTANT AWARDS AND THEIR FIELDS

Award	Field
Abel Prize	Mathematics
Aga Khan Award	Architecture
Arjuna Award	Sports and games
BAFTA Awards	Television, Films, Video Games and Animation
Bharat Ratna	Arts, Literature, Science and Public Service but the Government expanded the criteria to include "any field of human endeavor"
Booker Prize, Vyas Samman, Moorti Devi Award, Jnanpith Award, Saraswati Samman, Bihari Puraskar	Literature
Bowelay Award	Agriculture
Dadasaheb Phalke Award	Cinema
Dhanvantari Award	Medical Sciences
Dhyan Chand Award	Lifetime achievement in Sports and games
Dronacharya Award	Eminent Coaches of any particular sport
FiFi Awards	Fragrance Industry's creative achievements
Gallantry Awards: Paramvir Chakra Maha Vir Chakra Ashok Chakra Vir Chakra Shaurya Chakra	India's highest award for bravery Second highest gallantry award Highest peace-time gallantry award Third highest gallantry award For Bravery and gallant
Grammy Award	Music
Green Star Awards	Extraordinary efforts to respond to environmental disasters around the world
International Gandhi Peace Prize	Social, Economic and Political revolution through nonviolence and Gandhian Philosophy
Juliet Curie Award	Peace
Kalidas Samman	Classical Music and Dance
Kalinga Prize	Science
Lal Bahadur Shastri National Award	Public Administration, Management and Academics
Magsaysay Award	Outstanding contributions to Public service, Community Leadership, Journalism, Literature and Creative Arts and International Understanding
Manthan Award	e- Content and Creativity
Merlin	Magic
Nobel Prize	Achievements in the field of Physics, Chemistry, Peace, Economics, Medicine and Literature
Oscar Awards	Film Industry
Padma Awards	Exceptional and distinguished service in any field including service rendered by Government Servants

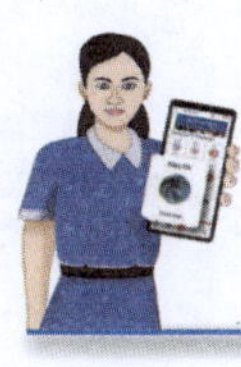

Contd...

Award	Field
Pritzker Prize	Architecture
Pulitzer Prize	Achievements in newspaper and online journalism, Literature, and musical composition in the United states
Right Livelihood Award	Environment and social Justice
Rajiv Gandhi Khel Ratna Award	Sports
Sahitya Akademi Award	Books in Indian Languages and English
Sangeet- Natak Akademi Award	Music, Drama and Dance
Shanti Swarup Bhatnagar Prize	Science and Technology
Stirling Prize	Architecture
Tansen Award	Music
UNESCO Human Rights Awards	Human Rights awareness
UNESCO Peace Prize	Contributions for International Peace
Vyas Samman	Hindi Literature
World Food Prize	Agriculture and Food Development

FAMOUS INDIAN CITIES AND THEIR NICKNAMES

State	City	Nickname
Andhra Pradesh	• Guntur • Kakinada • Rajahmundry • Tirupati • Vijayawada • Visakhapatnam	• City of Chillies • City of Kaja, Pensioners' Paradise • Cultural city • Spiritual Capital of Andhra Pradesh • The Place of victory • The City of destiny
Assam	• Dibrugarh • Guwahati • Tezpur	• Tea city of India • Gateway to the North-east India • The City of blood
Bihar	• Bhagalpur • Nalanda	• Silk City of India • The Land of knowledge
Chandigarh	• Chandigarh	• Beautiful City
Chhattisgarh	• Bhilai • Korba	• Steel Capital of India • Power Hub of India
Delhi	• New Delhi	• City of Rallies
Gujarat	• Karnavati (Ahmedabad) • Surat • Vadodara	• Boston of India/Manchester of India • Diamond City of India/Textile City of India • Cultural City of India/Sayaji Nagari/Banyan City/World capital of Garba
Haryana	• Bhiwani • Gurgaon • Panipat	• Mini Cuba • Millennium City of India • City of Weavers/City of Handloom
Jammu and Kashmir	• Kashmir • Srinagar	• Switzerland of India • City of Lakes
Jharkhand	• Dhanbad • Jamshedpur	• Coal Capital of India • Steel City/Pittsburgh of India
Karnataka	• Bengaluru • Coorg • Mangalore • Mysore	• Science City of India/Garden city of India/Silicon Valley of India/Space City • Scotland of India • Rome of the East/Cradle of Indian Banking • Heritage city of Karnataka/City of Palaces/Green City

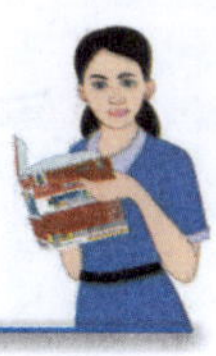

Contd...

State	City	Nickname
Kerala	• Kochi • Kollam • Kozhikode • Thrissur	• Queen of Arabian Sea/Gateway to Kerala • Cashew Capital of the World/Prince of Arabian Sea/Gateway of Backwater • City of Spices • Gold capital of India
Madhya Pradesh	• Bhopal • Indore • Ujjain	• City of Lakes • Mini Mumbai • City of Temples
Maharashtra	• Kolhapur • Mumbai • Nagpur • Nasik • Pune	• City of Wrestlers • Financial Capital of India/City of Seven Islands/City of Dreams • City of Oranges • Wine Capital of India/Grape City of India/California of India • Queen of Deccan
Meghalaya	• Shillong	• Scotland of the East
Nagaland	• Zunheboto	• Land of Warriors
Odisha	• Bhubaneswar • Cuttack • Rourkela	• Temple City of India • Silver City • Steel city of Odisha
Puducherry	• Puducherry	• Paris of the East
Punjab	• Ludhiana • Patiala	• Manchester of Punjab • Royal City
Rajasthan	• Jaipur • Jaisalmer • Jodhpur • Udaipur	• Pink City/Paris of India/City of Palaces • Golden City of India • Blue City/Sun City • Venice of the East/White city/City of Lakes
Tamil Nadu	• Chennai • Coimbatore • Kodaikanal • Madurai • Nilgiri • Ooty • Thiruchirappalli • Tirunelveli • Vaniyambadi	• Detroit of India/Auto Hub of India Health Capital of India/Gateway of South India • Manchester of South India/Textile City of India/Pump City • Princess of Hill stations • Athens of the East/City of Festivals/Temple city/Sleepless City/City of Four Junctions • Blue Mountain • Queen of Hill Stations • Rock Fort City/Tucker Trichy/Energy Equipment and fabrication capital of India • City of Paddy Fields/Oxford City of South India/Halwa City of India • Leather city of South India
Telangana	• Hyderabad • Warangal	• City of Pearls/HITECH City/City of Nizams/City of Biryani • City of Lakes/City of Temples/Second City of Nizam
Uttar Pradesh	• Agra • Kanpur • Lucknow • Prayagraj (Allahabad) • Varanasi	• City of Taj/Petha Nagri • Leather City of India/Manchester of North India • The Golden City of India/City of Nawabs/Constantinople of the East/Shiraz-e Hind • City of Prime Ministers/Sangam city/Abode of the God • The City of Light/Spiritual Capital of India/Oldest Living city on Earth/Holy City/City of Learning
Uttarakhand	• Mussoorie • Nainital • Rishikesh	• Queen of the Mountains • City of Lakes • Yoga capital of the world
West Bengal	• Asansol • Darjeeling • Durgapur • Kolkata • Malda • Purulia	• Land of Black Diamonds • Queen of Hills • Ruhr of India • City of Joy/Heaven of the Aged/Gateway of Eastern India • Mango City • Manbhum City

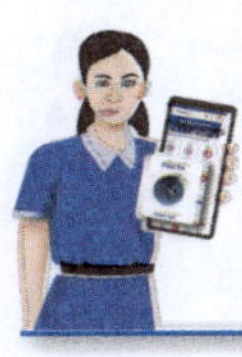

NOBEL PRIZE 2022

Sl. No.	Field	Winner	Contribution
1.	Physics	Alain Aspect, John F. Clauser, Anton Zeilinger	For experiments with entangled photons, establishing the violation of Bell inequalities and pioneering quantum information science
2.	Chemistry	Carolyn R. Bertozzi, Morten Meldal, K. Barry Sharpless	For the development of click chemistry and bioorthogonal chemistry
3.	Physiology or Medicine	Svante Pääbo	For his discoveries concerning the genomes of extinct hominins and human evolution
4.	Literature	Annie Ernaux	For the courage and clinical acuity with which she uncovers the roots, estrangements and collective restraints of personal memory
5.	Peace	Ales Bialiatski, Memorial, Center for Civil Liberties	The Peace Prize laureates represent civil society in their home countries. They have promoted the right to criticize power and protect the fundamental rights of citizens for many years. They have made an outstanding effort to document war crimes, human right abuses and the abuse of power. Together they demonstrate the significance of civil society for peace and democracy
6.	Economic Sciences	Ben S. Bernanke, Douglas W. Diamond, Philip H. Dybvig	For research on banks and financial crises

68TH FILMFARE AWARDS 2023

Sl. No.	Category	Winner
1.	Best Film	Gangubai Kathiawadi
2.	Best Film (Critics)	Badhaai Ho
3.	Best Actor Male	Rajkumar Rao (Badhaai Ho)
4.	Best Actor Female	Alia Bhatt (Gangubai Kathiawadi)
5.	Best Actor (Critics)	Sanjay Mishra (Vadh)
6.	Best Director	Sanjay Leela Bhansali (Gangubai Kathiawadi)
7.	Best Actor in Supporting Role (Male)	Anil Kapoor (Jug Jug Jeeyo)
8.	Best Actor in Supporting Role (Female)	Sheeba Chaddha (Baddhai Ho)
9.	Best Music album	Pritam for Brahmastra
10.	Best Dialogue	Prakash Kapadia and Utkarshini Vashistha for Gangubai Kathiawadi)
11.	Lifetime achievement award	Prem Chopra
12.	Best Playback Singer (Male)	Arjit Singh for Kesariya
13.	Best Playback Singer (Female)	Kavita Seth for Rangisari for Jug Jug Jeeyo

95TH ACADEMY AWARDS 2023

Sl. No.	Category	Winner
1.	Best Actor in leading role	BRENDAN FRASER (The Whale)
2.	Best Actor in supporting role	KE HUY QUAN (Everything Everywhere All at Once)
3.	Best Actress in leading role	MICHELLE YEOH (Everything Everywhere All at Once)
4.	Best Actress in supporting role	JAMIE LEE CURTIS (Everything Everywhere All at Once)
5.	Best Animated Feature Film	GUILLERMO DEL TORO'S PINOCCHIO (Guillermo del Toro, Mark Gustafson, Gary Ungar and Alex Bulkley)
6.	Best Direction	Daniel Kwan and Daniel Scheinert (Everything Everywhere All at Once)
7.	Best Documentary Feature Film	NAVALNY (Daniel Roher, Odessa Rae, Diane Becker, Melanie Miller and Shane Boris)
8.	Best International Feature Film	ALL QUIET ON THE WESTERN FRONT (Germany)
9.	Best Music	ALL QUIET ON THE WESTERN FRONT (Volker Bertelmann)
10.	Best Song	NAATU NAATU (From RRR; Music by M.M. Keeravaani; Lyric by Chandrabose)

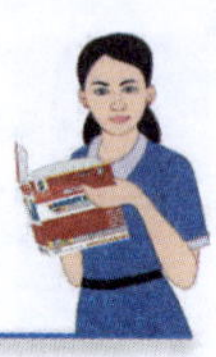

DADASAHEB PHALKE INTERNATIONAL FILM FESTIVAL 2023

Sl. No.	Category	Winner
1.	Best Film	The Kashmir Files
2.	Film of The Year	RRR
3.	Best Actor	Ranbir Kapoor (Brahmastra Part One: Shiva)
4.	Best Actress	Alia Bhatt (Gangubhai Kathiawadi)
5.	Critics Best Actor	Varun Dhawan (Bhediya)
6.	Critics Best Actress	Vidya Balan (Jalsa)
7.	Best Director	R Balki (Chup)
8.	Best Cinematographer	PS Vinod (Vikram Vedha)
9.	Most Promising Actor	Rishab Shetty (Kantara)
10.	Best Actor in a Supporting Role	Manish Paul (Jug Jug Jeeyo)
11.	Best Playback Singer (Male)	Sachet Tandon (Maiyya Mainu – Jersey)
12.	Best Playback Singer (Female)	Neeti Mohan (Meri Jaan – Gangubhai Kathiawadi)
13.	Best Web Series	Rudra: The Edge of Darkness (Hindi)
14.	Most Versatile Actor	Anupam Kher (The Kashmir Files)
15.	Television Series of The Year	Anupamaa
16.	Best Actor in a Television Series	Zain Imam for Fanaa (Ishq Mein Marjawaan)
17.	Best Actress in a Television Series	Tejasswi Prakash (Naagin)
18.	Dadasaheb Phalke International Film Festival Awards 2023 for Outstanding Contribution in the Film Industry	Rekha
19.	Dadasaheb Phalke International Film Festival Awards 2023 for Outstanding Contribution in the Music Industry	Hariharan

AWARDS AND RECOGNITION

Sl. No.	Awards	Awardee	Field
JUNE 2023			
1.	Gandhi Peace Prize	Gita Press Gorakhpur	For exceptional contribution to social, economic and political transformation through nonviolent and Gandhian methods
2.	Guinness World Record Award Certificate	Portuguese footballer Cristiano Ronaldo	For becoming the first men's player to make 200 international appearance
3.	Sahitya Akademi Bal Sahitya Puraskar 2023	Indian writer Priya AS	For Children's literature in Malayalam for her 2018 novel Perumazhayathe Kunjithalukal
4.	1st Kala Kranti Lifetime Achievement Award	Padma Shri Pandit Purna Das Baul	For his outstanding contribution to the traditional Baul music on the world stage
MAY 2023			
1.	British Academy of Film and Television Arts Fellowship (BAFTA)	Meera Syal	Outstanding and exceptional contribution to films, games and/or television
2.	2023 UNESCO/Guillermo Cano World Press Freedom Prize	Three imprisoned Iranian Journalists Niloofar Hamedi, Elaheh Mohammadi and Nargis Mohammadi	For exceptional contribution to the defense and/or advancement of press freedom worldwide

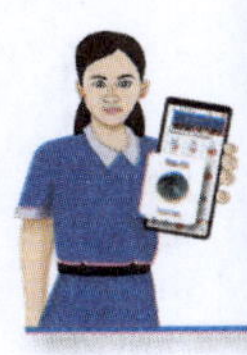

Contd...

Sl. No.	Awards	Awardee	Field
3.	Leipzig Book Award 2023	Russian poet Maria Stepanova	For her poetry entitled Mädchen ohne Kleider (Girls without Clothes)
4.	Bharat Ratna Dr Ambedkar Award	Yogi Adityanath, CM Uttar Pradesh	For creating fear free UP
5.	Laureus World Sportsman of the Year 2023	Lionel Messi (Argentine footballer)	For memorable sporting performance of 2022
6.	Pulitzer Prize 2023	Associated Press (American nonprofit news agency)	Journalism
7.	Chevalier de la Légion d'Honneur (Highest Civilian Honor)	N Chandrasekaran (Tata Sons chairman)	For his substantial role in developing and fostering commercial links between India and France
8.	International Booker Prize 2023	Georgi Gospodinov and translator Angela Rodel	For the dark comic Novel "Time Shelter"
APRIL 2023			
1.	Immigrant Achievement Awards	Neeli Bendapudi	Contribution to higher education in the US
2.	Global Gold Award	Power Grid Corporation of India Ltd (PGCIL)	Corporate social responsibility work
3.	Femina Miss India World 2023	Nandini Gupta	Beauty pageant winner
4.	Pravasi Bharatiya Samman Award	Raj Subramaniyam	Highest civilian recognition bestowed by India upon Indian descent and Indian diaspora
5.	Malcolm Adiseshiah Award 2023	Utsa Patnaik	Contribution to social science
6.	Lata Deenanath Mangeshkar Award	Asha Bhosle	Contribution to music
7.	Order of Merit	Angela Merkel	Contribution to German politics
8.	Excellence in Public Administration 2022	PM Gati Shakti National Master Plan	Innovative approach toward improving infrastructure
9.	Lifetime Achievement Award	Dr Raghu Ram Pillarisetti	Contribution to medicine
10.	Ramon Magsaysay Award	Dalai Lama	Leadership in safeguarding Tibetan religion and culture
11.	Order of Australia	Ratan Tata	Strengthening bilateral relationship between India and Australia
12.	Goldman Environmental Prize	Alessandra Korap	Efforts in Environmental Safeguarding
13.	Latin Women of the Year	Shakira	Contribution to Latin Music
MARCH 2023			
1.	Wildlife Conservation Award	Aliya Mir from Kashmir	For remarkable contribution to wildlife conservation
2.	SAARC Literary Award	Bangabandhu Sheikh Mujibur Rahman	Outstanding literary excellence in trilogy
3.	Abel Prize 2023	Luis Caffarelli	For his seminal contribution to regularity theory of nonlinear partial differential equation
4.	Saraswati Samman 2022	Sivasankari (Tamil writer)	For 2019 memoir Surya Vamsam
5.	Vyas Samman 2022	Gyan Chaturvedi	For Hindi novel Pagalkhana
6.	International Golden City Gate Tourism Awards 2023	Indian Ministry of Tourism and Government of India	For global effort on advertising the postcovid period to reopen opportunities in India
7.	Lifetime Achievement National Photography Award	Ms Sipra Das	Photographer in India

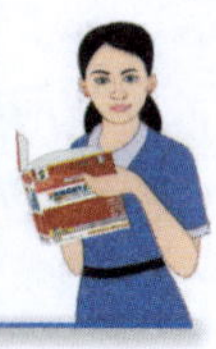

Contd...

Sl. No.	Awards	Awardee	Field
FEBRUARY 2023			
1.	Sangeet Natak Akademi Award 2019	Prem Kumar Mallick	For his contribution to the field of Hindustani Vocal Music
2.	Marconi Prize 2023	Hari Balakrishnan	For increasing digital inclusiveness through advanced information and communication technology
3.	Best Entrepreneur of the Year Award 2022	Indian Industrialist Sajjan Jindal	Best Entrepreneur
4.	National Geographic Picture of the Year	Karthik Subramaniam	Best picture of the year
5.	UNESCO Peace Prize	Angela Merkel	Outstanding contribution in the field of Human Rights and Peace Worldwide
6.	Raja Ram Mohan Roy National Award	ABK Prasad (Journalist)	For excellence in journalism
JANUARY 2023			
1.	Subhash Chandra Bose Disaster Management Award 2023	Odisha State Disaster Management Authority and Lunglei Fire Station Mizoram	For excellence in disaster management for the year 2023
2.	The most distinguished scientist of the year 2022	R Vishnu Prasad	For outstanding contribution in various fields, including culture, science, sports and innovation
3.	Miss Universe 2022	R'Bonney Gabriel (USA)	71st Miss Universe pageant
4.	Pravasi Bharatiya Samman Award 2023	Thiru Kumar Nadesan	For his contribution toward community welfare
5.	World Habitat Awards 2023 (UN Habitat's World)	Odisha	For Jaga mission, a land tilting and slum upgrading program
DECEMBER 2022			
1.	Atal Samman Award	Prabhu Chandra Mishra	Excellence in the field of science and research

AWARDS RECEIVED BY NARENDRA MODI TILL DATE

Country	Date	Note
Saudi Arabia	3rd April 2016	*Special Class*, the highest honor of Saudi Arabia awarded to non-Muslim dignitaries.
Afghanistan	4th June 2016	The highest civilian honor of Afghanistan.
Palestine	10th February 2018	The highest civilian honor of Palestine.
United Arab Emirates	4th April 2019	The highest civilian honor of the United Arab Emirates.
Russia	12th April 2019	The highest civilian honor of Russia.
Maldives	8th June 2019	The highest honor of the Maldives awarded to foreign dignitaries.
Bahrain	24th August 2019	First Class, the highest honor of Bahrain awarded to foreign dignitaries.
United States	21th December 2020	Chief Commander, the highest degree of the Legion of Merit.
Bhutan	17th December 2021	First Class, The highest civilian honor of Bhutan.
Fiji	22nd May 2023	Companion, the highest civilian honor of Fiji.
Papua New Guinea	22nd May 2023	Grand Companion, the highest civilian honor of Papua New Guinea.
Egypt	25th June 2023	Collar, the highest civilian honor of Egypt.
France	14th July 2023	Grand Cross, the highest civilian honor of France.

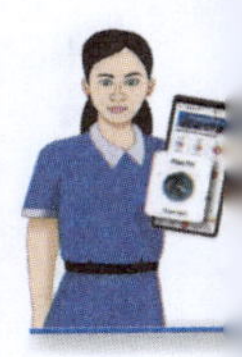

SPORTS

Sports Venue

Sports events	Venue
Asia Cup 2023	Pakistan and Sri Lanka
Men's Junior Asia Cup 2023	Oman
FIBA 3 x 3 World Cup World Cup 2023	Dubai
2023 Asia U20 Athletics Championship	South Korea
Special Olympics World Summer Games 2023	Germany
2023 World Table Tennis Championships	South Korea
2023 Women's Junior Asia Cup 2023	Argentina
UEFA EURO 2024	Germany

GRAND SLAMS

Four Grand Slams Timing and Courts

1. **Australian open:** Hard courts (Mid January)
2. **French Open (also known as Roland Garros):** Clay Court (late May to early June)
3. **Wimbledon (also known as UK Open):** Grass Courts (June–July)
4. **US Open- August:** Hard courts (September)

List of Winners of All Four Grand Slams

French Open 2023

Title	Winner	Runner-up
Men's Singles	Novak Djokovic (Serbia) 23rd Title	Casper Ruud
Women's Singles	Iga Świątek (Poland)	Karolina Muchova
Men's doubles	Ivan Dodig and Austin Krajicek	Sander Gille and Joran Vliegen
Women's doubles	Hsieh Su-Wei and Wang Xinyu	Taylor Towsend and Leylah Fernandez
Mixed doubles	Miyu Kato and Tim Pütz	Bianca Andreescu and Michael Venus

Australian Open 2023

Event	Winner	Runner-up
Men's Singles	Novak Djokovic (Serbia)	Stefanos Tsitsipas (Greece)
Women's Singles	Arina Sabalenka (Belarus)	Elena Rybakina (Kazakhstan)
Men's Doubles	J. Kubler and R. Hijikata (Australia)	H. Nys (Monaco) and J. Zieliński (Poland)
Women's Doubles	Barbora Krejčíková (Czech) Kateřina Siniaková (Czech)	S. Aoyama and E. Shibahara (Japan)
Mix Doubles	Luisa Stefani and Rafael Matos (Brazilian)	Rohan Bopanna and Sania Mirza (India)

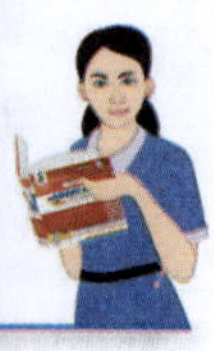

US Open 2022

Category	Winner	Runner-up
Men's singles	C. Alcaraz Garfia (Spain)	C. Ruud (Norway)
Women's singles	Iga Świątek (Poland)	O. Jabeur (Tunisia)
Men's doubles	R. Ram and J. Salisbury	W. Koolhof and N. Skupski
Women's doubles	K. Siniaková and B. Krejčíková	C. McNally and T. Townsend
Women's doubles	S. Sanders and J. Peers	K. Flipkens and É. Roger-Vasselin

Wimbledon 2023

Category	Winner	Runner-up
Men's Single	Carlos Alcaraz (Spain)	Novak Djokovic
Women's Single	Marketa Vondrousova (Czech Republic)	Ons Jabeur

Sports Events

Months	Sports Events
July 2023	Shah Rukh Khan appointed as the Brand Ambassador of ICC World Cup 2023
	Aditya Samant became India's 83rd Grandmaster
	West Indies failed to qualify for World Cup 2023
June 2023	The 2024 Olympics will be held in Paris, France from July 26 to Aug 11
	Cristiano Ronaldo set a Guinness World Record by Achieving 200 international caps for Portugal
May 2023	Satwiksairaj Rankireddy and Chirag Shetty created history by becoming the first Indian men's doubles pair to win a Gold Medal at the Badminton Asia Championship
	Shooters Mairaj Ahmad Khan and Ganemat Sekhon have won India the first medal in the ongoing International Shooting Sport Federation (ISSF) Shotgun World Cup in Cairo, Egypt
	Vankita Agarwal is the new Indian Woman No 3 in chess and the 11th Indian Woman to achieve the International Master Title
April 2023	On the occasion of 50th Birthday, Indian Cricket icon Sachin Tendulkar was honored in a special program held in the UAE where the West Stand at the Sharjah Cricket Stadium was renamed after him
March 2023	Virat Kohli has surpassed legendary West Indies Brian Lara to become the second highest run scorer against Australia in International Cricket
February 2023	The Australian Women's Cricket team has won the ICC World Cup Trophy 2023
January 2023	The 5th Edition of Khelo India Youth Games 2023 began in Bhopal, Madhya Pradesh
	The mascot of Khelo India Youth Game is Asha, while the theme song is "Hindustan ka Dil Dhadka Do"

List of ICC Awards Winner for 2022

- Men's Test Cricketer of the Year: Ben Stokes (England)
- Men's ODI Cricketer of the Year: Babar Azam (Pakistan)
- Women's ODI Cricketer of the Year: Nat Sciver (England)
- Men's T20 International Cricketer of the Year: Surya Kumar Yadav (India)
- Women's T20 International Cricketer of the Year: Tahila McGrath (Australia)
- Men's Emerging Cricketer of the Year: Marco Jansen (South Africa)
- Women's Emerging Cricketer of the Year: Renuka Singh (India)
- Spirit of Cricket Award: Ashif Seikh (Nepal)

Men's Hockey World Cup

- Best Player: Niklas Wellen (Germany)
- Best Goalkeeper: Vincent Vanasch (Belgium)
- Hero Top Scorer: Jeremy Hayward (Australia)
- Best Team Goal Celebration Award: Korea
- Maximum Team Goal Awards: Netherlands
- Best Defender of the tournament award: Jeremy Hayward (Australia)

PERSON IN NEWS

Constitutional Office Holders

Office	Name
President	Droupadi Murmu
Vice President and ex-officio Chairperson, Rajya Sabha	Jagdeep Dhankhar
Prime Minister	Narendra Modi
Chief Justice	Dhananjaya Y. Chandrachud
Speaker, Lok Sabha	Om Birla
Chief Election Commissioner	Rajiv Kumar
Comptroller and Auditor General	Girish Chandra Murmu
Chairperson, Union Public Service Commission	Dr Manoj Soni
Attorney General	R. Venkataramani

Heads of Important National Institutions

Important National Institution	Head
Chief of Defense Staff	General Anil Chauhan
Chief of the Army Staff	General Manoj Pandey
Chief of the Naval Staff	Admiral Radhakrishnan Hari Kumar
Chief of the Air Staff	Air Chief Marshal Vivek Ram Chaudhari
Director CBI	Praveen Sood
Director IB	Tapan Deka
National Human Rights Commission	Arun Kumar Mishra
National Commission for Backward Classes	Hansraj Gangaram Ahir
National Commission for Minorities	Iqbal Singh Lalpura
National Commission for Scheduled Tribes	Harsh Chouhan
National Commission for Scheduled Castes	Vijay Sampla
Indian Space Research Organization	Sreedhara Somanath
Atomic Energy Commission	Dr Ajit Kumar Mohanty
Securities and Exchange Board of India	Madhabi Puri Buch
Telecom Regulatory Authority of India (TRAI)	Ram Sewak Sharma
Central Board of Film Certification	Prasoon Joshi

Contd...

Important International Officials

Institution	Head
United Nations Organization (UNO)	António Guterres
World Bank	Ajay Banga
International Monetary Fund	Kristalina Georgieva
World Trade Organization	Dr Ngozi Okonjo-Iweala
The United Nations Educational, Scientific and Cultural Organization (UNESCO)	Audrey Azoulay
International Labor Organization	Gilbert F. Houngbo
World Health Organization (WHO)	Dr Tedros Adhanom Ghebreyesus
International Court of Justice	Joan E. Donoghue
UN Human Rights Council	Václav Bálek
North Atlantic Treaty Organization (NATO)	Jens Stoltenberg
Association of Southeast Asian Nations (ASEAN)	Kao Kim Hourn
South Asian Association for Regional Cooperation (SAARC)	Esala Weerakoon
Commonwealth	Charles III
Red Cross	Gail J. McGovern
Food and Agriculture Organization (FAO)	Qu Dongyu

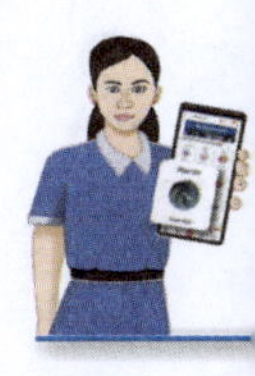

Companies and their CEOs

Company	CEO
Google	Sundar Pichai
Meta (Previously Facebook)	Mark Zuckerberg
Instagram	Adam Mosseri
Reliance Industry Limited	Mukesh Ambani/chairman, managing director, and largest shareholder
Infosys	NR Narayan Murthy/Chairman
Bharti Enterprises (Airtel)	Sunil Mittal

Heads of Financial and Sports Institutions

Institution	Head
Reserve Bank of India	Shaktikanta Das
Federation of Indian Chambers of Commerce and Industry (FICCI)	Mr Subhrakant Panda
National Bank for Agriculture and Rural Development (NABARD)	Shri Shaji K V
Small Industries Development Bank of India (SIDBI)	Shri Sivasubramanian Ramann
National Housing Bank	Shri Sarada Kumar Hota
The Associated Chambers of Commerce and Industry of India (ASSOCHAM)	Ajay Singh
International Chamber of Commerce	María Fernanda Garza
International Olympic Committee (IOC)	Thomas Bach (President)
The Fédération Internationale de Football Association (FIFA)	Gianni Infantino (President)
International Cricket Council (ICC)	Greg Barclay (Chairman)
International Hockey Federation (FIH)	Tayyab Ikram (President)
The International Association of Athletics Federations (IAAF)	Sebastian Coe (President)
International Tennis Federation (ITF)	David Haggerty (President)
Indian Olympic Association	PT Usha
All India Football Federation	Kalyan Chaubey (President)
Board of Control for Cricket in India (BCCI)	Roger Binny (President)
Hockey India	Dilip Tirkey (President)

Republic Day 2023

Egypt's President Abdel Fattah el-Sisi I was the Chief Guest on 74th Republic Day of India, January 2023.

LIST OF NATIONAL HEALTH PROGRAMMES IN INDIA

National Health Programmes	Year of Launch	Objective/Description
National Cancer Control Programme	1975	Primary prevention of cancers by health education regarding hazards of tobacco consumption and necessity of genital hygiene for prevention of cervical cancer, etc.
National Programme for Prevention and Control of Deafness (NPPCD)	2006– 2008	To prevent the avoidable hearing loss on account of disease or injury, etc.
District Mental Health Programme (DMHP)	1982	To ensure availability and accessibility of minimum mental health care for all in the foreseeable future, particularly to the most vulnerable and underprivileged sections of population.

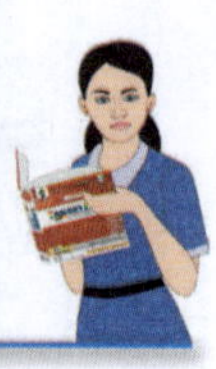

Contd...

National Health Programmes	Year of Launch	Objective/Description
National Cancer Registry Programme	1982	To provide true information on cancer prevalence and incidence.
National Leprosy Eradication Programme	Started in 1955, launched in 1983	To arrest the disease activity in all the known cases of leprosy.
Universal Immunization Programme (UIP)	1985	To achieve self-sufficiency in vaccine production and the manufacture of cold-chain equipment for storage purpose, etc.
National Vector Borne Disease Control Programme	----	For the prevention and control of vector borne diseases
National Tobacco Control Programme	2007	Preventing the initiation of smoking among young people, educating, motivating and assisting smokers to quit smoking, etc.
National Programme for Health Care of the Elderly (NPHCE)	2010	To provide preventive, curative and rehabilitative services to the elderly persons at various levels of health care delivery system of the country, etc.

NATIONAL HEALTH PROGRAMMES

1. **National Vector Borne Disease Control Programme (NVBDCP):** National Vector Borne Disease Control Programme (NVBDCP) is an umbrella program for prevention and control of six vector borne diseases, **viz., Malaria, Japanese Encephalitis (JE), Dengue, Chikungunya, Kala-Azar and Lymphatic Filariasis**. In UT of J&K, Malaria Annual Parasite Index (API) is 0.003, which is better than the national average. Major activities are, making blood smear of all cure cases, examination for Malarial parasite, antilarval measures and fogging during rainy season. In Dengue cases, this program ensures providing laboratory facilities for diagnosis of Dengue and its treatment.
2. **National Viral Hepatitis Control Programme (NVHCP):** Was launched by MoH&FW, GOI in July 2018 with an aim to eliminate Hepatitis C by 2030, to achieve significant reduction in infected population and morbidity associated with Hepatitis B & C. The UT of J&K has established two Model Treatment Centers in Department of Gastroenterology at GMC, Jammu/ GMC, Srinagar and 20 District Level Treatment Centers in District Hospitals under NVHCP. Moreover, J&K has designated two Referral Labs. Deptt. of Microbiology, GMC, Jammu & Deptt. of Microbiology, GMC, Srinagar and 20 District Laboratories under NVHCP. Viral Hepatitis Division, MoH&FW, GOI is supplying various drugs under NVHCP for treatment of Hepatitis B & C patients and same is being distributed to Model Treatment Centers and District Treatment Centers.
3. **National TB Elimination Programme (NTEP):** The program is implemented by Directorate of Health Services through State TB Officer at Division level and District TB Officer at District Level. The target under this program is to eliminate TB by 2025. Chest Disease (CD) Hospital, Jammu and CD Hospital, Srinagar are two major hospitals providing treatment to TB patients. All the diagnosis, i.e., Direct Microscopy, X-rays, CBNAAT/TRUNAT tests are free of cost. Diagnosed TB patients are provided with free medicines and nutritional support under NPY (Nikshay Poshan Yojana) @ ₹500 per month for treatment. The status of all TB patients with regard to diabetes and HIV is also provided. TB Elimination programme is one of the priority areas of GOI and UT Govt. In UT of J&K, District Budgam is declared as TB free in 2020–21, District Anantnag, Pulwama, Kupwara got gold medal and District Baramulla got Bronze medal for Subnational Certification by GoI.
4. **National Leprosy Eradication Programme (NLEP):** National Leprosy Eradication Programme was introduced in 1983. The NLEP's mission is to provide quality leprosy services free of cost to all the sections of population, with easy accessibility, through the integrated health care system, including care for disability cure of the disease. NLEP programme is funded by NHM and implemented by concerned Directorate through Zonal Leprosy Officer at Divisional level and supported by *District.* The main services provided are Information Education and Communication (IEC) for creating awareness about Leprosy, its preventive measures and treatment facilities. The active case finding survey – **Sparsh** is conducted in areas prone to Leprosy. The treatment of Leprosy is free of cost.
5. **National Rabies Control Programme (NRCP):** NRCP has been approved under 12th Five-Year Plan, it has both human and animal health components. The target of NRCP is that there should be no case of death due to rabies by 2030. Under this program, Anti Rabies Serum (ARS) and Anti Rabies Vaccine (ARV) is provided to Dog bite/Animal bite victim. The treatment is free of cost and it is funded by NHM. Under the program Model, Rabies Centers are established (i) at GMC-Jammu and (ii) at GMC- Srinagar.
6. **Integrated Disease Surveillance Programme (IDSP)-IHIP:** Integrated Disease Surveillance Programme is a decentralized, State based Surveillance Program. It is intended to detect early warning signals of impending outbreaks and helps to initiate an effective response in a timely manner. It aims to strengthen/ maintain decentralized laboratory based IT enabled disease surveillance system for epidemic prone diseases and to detect and respond to outbreaks in early rising phase through trained Rapid Response Teams (RRTs). Whenever, there is a rising trend of illnesses in any area, it is investigated by the RRTs established in all districts to diagnose and control the outbreak. Data analysis and actions are to be undertaken by State/District Surveillance Units. Initially, IDSP Portal was designed for weekly based reporting of data on portal with monitoring of only 13 health conditions.

   In UT J&K, Integrated Health Information Platform (IHIP) was launched in April, 2021 and reporting was started, on

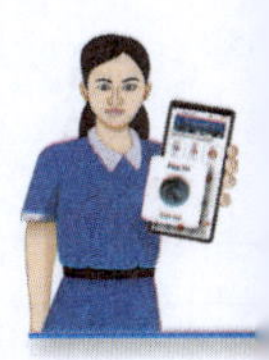

1st October 2021. The complete migration from old portal to IHIP Portal was done and old IDSP portal was stopped for reporting, Presently, IHIP is the reporting Portal of IDSP.

7. **102–108 (JKEMS) Ambulance Services:** 102–108 Ambulance Service under J&K Emergency Medical Services, an initiative of NHM, was launched on 24th March, 2020 in the Union Territory of J&K by the then Hon'ble Lieutenant Governor, Sh. G.C Murmu. The service provides Emergency Medical Services, with immediate response and dispatch of Ambulance to the site of emergency, after the call has been received on Toll Free Numbers 108 & 102. Emergency Medical Response Service (EMS) is specialized field where emergency health care needs are addressed through well-defined care processed by trained EMS professionals. The important aspect of Emergency response includes early detection of any emergency, immediate response, on-scene care, en-route care and transfer of the victim to health care facility. There is greater need to standardize ambulances and professional education for effective delivery of Comprehensive Emergency Medical Response Service.

8. **National Tobacco Control Programme (NTCP):** Tobacco is the leading global cause of preventable death. It kills nearly 6 million people and causes hundreds of billions of dollars of economic damage worldwide each year. Most of these deaths occur in low and middle income countries, and this disparity is expected to widen further over the next several decades. However, a substantial development took place in 2003 with the unanimous adoption of WHO Framework Convention on Tobacco Control (WHO-FCTC). A number of countries have legislation restricting tobacco advertising and regulating who can buy and use tobacco products, and where people can smoke. India has also enacted the tobacco control legislation namely, "The Cigarettes and other Tobacco Products (Prohibition of Advertisement and Regulation of Trade and Commerce, Production, Supply and Distribution) Act" in the year 2003.

   Further, India is one of the first few countries to have dedicated National Tobacco Control Programme (NTCP). In September 2011, the global tobacco control movement took on new prominence as global leaders came together in New York for the first ever United Nations High-Level Meeting on Noncommunicable Diseases (NCDs). At this historic gathering, world leaders unanimously approved an action plan for combating NCDs that has the potential to meaningfully impact the tobacco epidemic. This plan calls for greater international collaboration and for programs that help combat tobacco.

   These milestones are impressive, so are the challenges and opportunities ahead. With cross sector commitment and collaboration, millions of lives can be saved by preventing tobacco related deaths. Effective tobacco control, more than anything else, can substantially help reduce the toll of NCDs and prevent related deaths. National Tobacco Control Programme (NTCP) is implemented in all Districts of the UT of J&K through both the Directorates of Health Services.

9. **Biomedical Equipment Management and Maintenance Program (BEMMP):** Biomedical Equipment Management and Maintenance Program is an initiative by 'Ministry of Health and Family Welfare, Government of India' through 'National Health Mission' to provide support to state Governments to outsource medical equipment maintenance comprehensively for all facilities, so as to improve the functionality and life of equipment, simultaneously improving health care services in public health facilities, reducing cost of care and improving the quality of care. On behalf of Government of J&K, JK Medical Supplies Cooperation (JKMSCL) has signed the MOU with M/s Mediciti, Health Care Services, Pvt., Ltd. for a period of 5 years on PPP mode and which is extendable for another term of 5 years (based on performance) with Mediciti on PPP mode. The Project was started on 18th of November 2019 across the UT of J&K (These include all the District Hospitals, Sub-District Hospitals / Community Health Centers, and PHCs Level).

10. **National Programme for Prevention and Control of Cancer, Diabetes, Cardiovascular Diseases and Stroke (NPCDCS):** In order to prevent and control major Noncommunicable Diseases, National Programme for Prevention and Control of Cancer, Diabetes, Cardiovascular Diseases and Stroke was launched in 2010 with focus on strengthening infrastructure, human resource development, health promotion, early diagnosis, management and referral. Under NPCDCS, NCD Cells are being established at National, State and District levels for Programme Management, and NCD Clinics are being set up at District and CHC levels, to provide services for early diagnosis, treatment and follow-up for common NCDs. Provision has been made under the program to provide free diagnostic facilities and drugs for patients attending the NCD clinics. Cardiac Care Units (CCU) are also being set up in identified Districts for providing facilities for emergency Cardiac Care. Day Care Centers at the identified districts are set up to provide facilities for Cancer care. In J&K, Screening for Diabetes, Hypertension and three major cancers is done at Health and Wellness Center (HWCs) and uploaded on NCD Portal.

11. **National Quality Assurance Standards (NQAS):** National Quality Assurance Standards have been developed keeping in the specific requirements for public health facilities as well as global best practices. NQAS are currently available for District Hospitals, CHCs, PHCs and Urban PHCs. Standards are primarily meant for providers to assess their own quality for improvement through pre-defined standards and to bring up their facilities for certification. The National Quality Assurance Standards are broadly arranged under 8 "Areas of Concern"– Service Provision, Patient Rights, Inputs, Support Services, Clinical Care, Infection Control, Quality Management and Outcome. These standards are ISQUA accredited and meet global benchmarks in terms of comprehensiveness, objectivity, evidence and rigor of development.

12. **Kayakalp:** Clean environment improves healing and fastens recovery, besides enhancing patients' experience at health facility. The Union Health and Family Welfare Minister Shri J P Nadda has launched 'Kayakalp Award Scheme' on May 15, 2015 as an extension of 'Swachh Bharat Mission'. Aim of initiative was to improve and promote the cleanliness, hygiene, waste management and infection control practices in public health care facilities and incentivize the exemplary performing facilities. The objectives of the award scheme are:
    - To inculcate a culture of ongoing assessment and peer review of performance related to hygiene, sanitation and infection control.

- To incentivize and recognize public health care facilities that show exemplary performance in adhering to standard protocols of cleanliness, infection control and sanitation,
- To create and share sustainable practices related to improving cleanliness in public health facilities which lead to positive health outcomes.

13. **Rashtriya Kishor Swasthya Karyakram (RKSK):** In order to ensure holistic development of adolescent population, the Ministry of Health and Family Welfare launched Rashtriya Kishor Swasthya Karyakram (RKSK) on 7th January 2014 to reach out to 253 million adolescents—male and female, rural and urban, married and unmarried, in and out-of-school adolescents with special focus on marginalized and undeserved groups.
14. **Menstrual Hygiene Scheme (MHS):** The Ministry of Health and Family Welfare has introduced a scheme for promotion of menstrual hygiene among adolescent girls in the age group of 10–19 years in rural areas. The major objectives of the schemes are (i) to increase awareness among adolescent girls on Menstrual Hygiene (ii) to increase access to and use of high quality sanitary napkins to adolescent girls in rural areas.
15. **Mera Asptaal (MA):** Mera Aspataal (My Hospital) is a Ministry of Health and Family Welfare, Government of India (GOI) initiative to capture patient's feedback on the services received from both public and empanelled private health facilities. It works through multiple communication channels, including Short Message Service (SMS), Outbound Dialing (OBD), a mobile application, and a web portal. The application allows feedback to be consolidated, analyzed and disseminated on a frequently updated dashboard. Analyzed data will be used to improve quality of services in health care facilities. Thus, My Hospital aligns with the citizen centric MyGov platform of GOI which allows patients to connect with the health care providers and policymakers and to have their opinion heard and acted upon.
16. **Pradhan Mantri National Dialysis Programme (PMNDP):** The Pradhan Mantri National Dialysis Programme (PMNDP) aims at strengthening of District Hospitals by providing affordable dialysis services. In J&K, all 20 District hospitals are having operational dialysis units to implement this program.
17. **NHM Free Diagnostics Service Initiative:** Government of India under the National Health Mission launched the Free Essential Diagnostics Initiative to address the high, out of pocket expenditure on diagnostics. The objective of the Free Diagnostic Services Initiative program is to ensure availability and access to diagnostic tests at public health facilities so as to reduce out of pocket expenditure incurred by patients on diagnostics. Provision of appropriate diagnostics is necessary and critical in providing adequate comprehensive health care services in public health facilities. In UT J&K free drugs and diagnostics initiative program is functional in HWCs only.
18. **Drugs and Vaccine Distribution Management System (DVDMS):** It is a software platform to automate various activities of Directorate General Medical Health, Ministry of health and family welfare Govt. of India. It comprises Drug and Vaccine Supply Chain Management that deals with Purchase Order, Inventory Management & Distribution of various drugs, etc. In J&K, DVDMS is funded by NHM and is operational by J&K Medical Supplies Corporation Ltd.
19. **National Programme on Climate Change & Human Health (NPCCHH):**
    The program aims:
    - To create awareness among general population (vulnerable community), health care providers and policy makers regarding impacts of climate change on human health.
    - To strengthen capacity of health care system to reduce illnesses/ diseases due to variability in climate.
    - To strengthen health preparedness and response by performing situational analysis at national/state/district/ below district levels.
    - To develop partnerships and create synchrony/synergy with other missions and ensure that health is adequately represented in the climate change agenda in the country.
    - To strengthen research capacity to fill the evidence gap on climate change impact on human health. In J&K, UT Organizing Committee state task force and environmental cells have been officially framed by General Administration Department, J&K. ARI surveillance is being carried on in three sentinel Hospitals in Jammu City.
20. **Maternal Health**
    - **Janani Suraksha Yojana (JSY):** In order to promote safe institutional deliveries, the Govt. of India has implemented JSY throughout the country including Jammu and Kashmir. The JSY is being implemented in all Govt. Hospitals of the state to enable increase in number of institutional deliveries and reduce maternal, infant mortality and in particular neonatal mortality by promoting institutional delivery among the needy and poor pregnant women of rural and urban areas. The JSY is being implemented in the State since 2005-06. The JSY benefits to the mother are being paid after the delivery and before the discharge, but not later than 7 days of delivery. In case of referrals, the payment is made within 15 days of delivery. All the payments are being made through DBT mode of payment. Under this scheme, the incentives are being paid to mother beneficiaries at the following norms:

Sl. No.	Area	Incentive for mother beneficiary
1.	Rural areas	₹1400.00
2.	Urban areas	₹1000.00
3.	BPL mothers delivering at home	₹500.00

ASHAs will facilitate antenatal checkups and accompany the mothers to the health institutions for delivery and will get the following incentives:

Sl. No.	Area	Incentive for ASHA
1.	Rural areas	₹600.00 (For facilitating full ANC and institutional delivery)
2.	Urban areas	₹400.00 (For facilitating full ANC and institutional delivery)

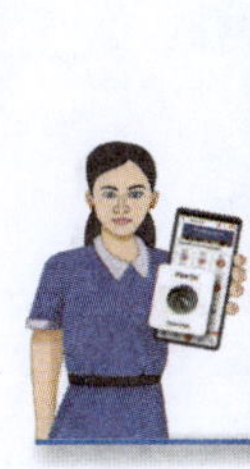

- **Janani Shishu Suraksha Karyakram (JSSK):** With the launch of the Janani Suraksha Yojana (JSY), the number of institutional deliveries has increased significantly. There are however, about 15 to 20% pregnant women who still hesitate to access public health facilities. Those who have opted for institutional delivery are not willing to stay for 48 hours, hampering the provision of essential services both to the mother and neonates, which are critical for identification and management of complications during the first 48 hours after delivery. To encourage women to stay for 48 hours at the facility after delivery and to make zero out of pocket expenditure, Janani Shishu Suraksha Karyakram (JSSK) has been implemented in the State vide Govt. Order No. 516-HME of 2011 since October 2011, with a view to encourage all pregnant women to deliver in Public Health Facilities and fulfill the commitment of achieving cent percent institutional deliveries. JSSK aims at mitigating the burden of out of pocket expenses incurred by families of pregnant women and sick infants, and acts as a major factor in enhancing access to public health institutions and helps in bringing down the Maternal and Infant Mortality. The entitlements under the program for Pregnant

  Women & Infants are:

  1. Free and zero expense treatment.
  2. Free drugs and consumables.
  3. Free diagnostics.
  4. Free diet to mothers during hospital stay.
  5. Free provision of blood, preferably on replacement basis.
  6. Free transport from home to health institution, between health institutions in case of referrals and drop back home.
  7. Exemption from all kinds of user charges.

- **Maternal Death Surveillance & Response (MDSR):** Maternal Death Review (MDR) strategy has been implemented in the State since 2011-12 to analyze various factors responsible for maternal deaths at community level as well as at facility level. It is an important strategy to improve the quality of obstetric care and reduce maternal mortality and morbidity. The importance of MDR lies in the fact that it provides detailed information on various factors at facility, district, community, regional and national level that are needed to be addressed to reduce maternal deaths. Analysis of these deaths can identify the delays that contribute to maternal deaths at various levels and the information used to adopt measures to fill the gaps in service.

  At the District level, the Maternal Death Review is envisaged at two levels.

  1. Maternal Death Review under chairmanship of CMO.
  2. Maternal Death Review by District Level Committee under chairmanship of District Magistrate.

  Composition of District Level Committee

District magistrate	Chairperson
Chief Medical Officer	Member Secretary/ Convener
Dy. Chief Medical Officer	Member
District Nodal Officer (MDR)	Member
Facility Based Nodal Officer (MDR)	Member
Representative of Federation of Obstetric and Gynecological Society of India (FOGSI)	Member

Contd...

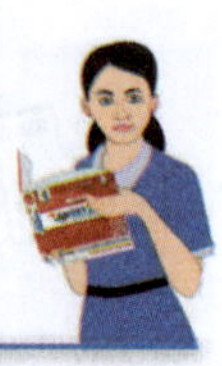

- **Pradhan Mantri Surakshit Matritva Abhiyan (PMSMA):** With an objective to provide quality ANC to every pregnant woman, the Government of India has launched the "Pradhan Mantri Surakshit Matritva Abhiyan". ANCs are given a fixed day, **on 9th of every month** across the country, where pregnant women will get antenatal care services by Specialists and Medical Officers at the PHC/CHC/DH levels. This is to be given in addition of the routine ANC at the health facility. If the 9th day of the month is a Sunday/ a holiday, then the services shall be provided on the next working day.

  This new initiative was rolled out in Jammu and Kashmir on **9th June, 2016** in all the districts of the state. Under this campaign, a minimum package of antenatal care services would be provided to beneficiaries on the 9th day of every month at health facilities to ensure that every pregnant woman receives at least one checkup in the 2nd and 3rd trimester of pregnancy and to ensure that no high risk pregnancy goes undetected.

  During this campaign, trained service providers and ASHAs will focus their efforts to identify and reach out to pregnant women who are not registered for ANC (left out/ missed ANC) and also those who are registered but those who did not avail ANC services (dropout) as well as High Risk pregnant women. It will also be ensured that not only all pregnant women complete their scheduled ANC visits, but also undertake all essential investigations. While 9th of every month will be organized as a special day, it is reiterated that the existing, routine and planned services such as ANC, PNC, etc. will continue to be delivered at all the facilities as scheduled in their respective microplans.

- **Surakshit Matritva Aashwasan (SUMAN):** Under SUMAN, all existing initiatives for strengthening Maternal and Child Health like JSY, JSSK, PMSMA, MDSR, LaQshya, FBNC, HBNC, HBYC have been subsumed under one umbrella in order to create a comprehensive initiative which goes beyond entitlements and provides assured service guarantee for the entitlements. In this regard, Govt. of J&K, GAD Deptt. has constituted Committees at Union Territory level, District Level and Block Level for implementation of SUMAN vide Govt. order no 688-JK(GAD) of 2021 dated 05-08-2021. To ensure implementation of key activities under SUMAN initiative, sanction is accorded to notification of SUMAN CEMONC, SUMAN BEMONC and SUMAN basic facilities vide Govt. order no 683-JK(HME) of 2021 dated 27-10-2021 issued by Health & Medical Education Department, J&K.

- **Establishment of Obstetric ICU at Medical Colleges:** For management of high risk pregnancies who have progressed to a clinical condition where there is multi-organ involvement/ failure, thus requiring vigilant monitoring and interventions by specially trained teams, 4 bedded Obstetric ICUs have been established, one each at SMGS Hospital, Jammu & LD Hospital Srina,gar under NHM, for providing quality care during obstetric and gynecological emergencies.

21. **ASHA Programme:** ASHA (Accredited Social Health Activist) is a band of female health volunteers which has been created as one of the key components of the National Health Mission. She is a trained female health activist in the community to create awareness on health and mobilizes the community toward local health planning, increased utilization of health services so as to increase accountability of the health service providers. The ASHA Programme has been implemented in all 20 districts and 109 blocks of the UT with about 816 ASHA clusters being developed for better management of the program.

The ASHA Facilitators, Block ASHA Coordinators & District ASHA Coordinators are the ASHA Cadres and they are the officials of permanent cadres of Health Department, for mentoring and monitoring at Cluster, Block, and District level respectively.

Social Security Schemes of ASHAs

- NHM, J&K is providing various social security schemes to the ASHAs of J&K:
- NHM, J&K shall be paying compensation to the family if an ASHA suffers loss of life or is permanently disabled, or is suffering from a life-threatening condition.
- In case of permanent disability to an ASHA due to any natural or unnatural cause, she will be paid lumpsum amount of ₹2.5 lakhs.
- If an ASHA suffers from loss of life, the legal dependent of the deceased will be paid lumpsum amount one time ₹5 lakhs.
- She shall also be getting financial assistance of up to ₹2 lakhs for grave health conditions requiring medical interventions.

22. **DNB Courses Under NBE in UT of J&K:** National Board of Examinations (NBE), established by the Government of India has been improving the quality of Medical Education by establishing high and uniform standards of postgraduate examinations in modern medicine on All India basis. NBE conducts postgraduate and postdoctoral examinations in approved disciplines leading to the award of Diplomate of National Board (DNB) and Fellow of National Board (FNB).

DNB Courses have been initiated in the District Hospitals of UT of J&K in 2019–20, keeping in view the urgent need of strengthening the District Hospitals, thereby enhancing the scope of specialized clinical services, teaching & research in the District Hospitals. This could also generate significant amount, additional revenue and decongest the tertiary care facilities to a larger extent.

Benefits:

- Additional Manpower especially the availability of Specialists at District implementing DNB.
- Decongestion of Govt. Medical Colleges.
- Reduction in referral from the facilities to tertiary care institutes.
- There will be strengthening of the peripheral care facilities.
- The institution will get 10% extra on every identified package over and above which is allowed under individual packages under Ayushman Bharat Yojana.
- The Districts applying for DNB courses have to qualify for NQAS also and get 25% incentive from the Ministry of Health & Family Welfare, Govt. of India.
- There will be opportunities for Medical professionals for research, training and teaching experiences.
- The institution (DH/ CHC) shall become a teaching hospital.

- **Health & Wellness Centers (H&WC):** Provision of Comprehensive Primary Health Care is an integral and pivotal part of Universal Health Coverage (UHC) and there is felt need of generating evidence to evolve innovative solutions for strengthening the Primary Health care. Comprehensive Primary Health Care includes the delivery of a package of primitive, curative and rehabilitative services delivered close to communities by Health care providers.
- **Rashtriya Bal Swasthya Karyakram (RBSK):** Rashtriya Bal Swasthya Karyakram (RBSK) is another initiative of MoH&FW, GoI under National Health Mission which aims at screening children from 0 to 18 years of age for Ds- Defects, Deficiencies and Development delays including Disabilities. Children diagnosed with these defects/diseases shall receive free of cost treatment including surgical interventions and follow-up at tertiary level under this program. The objective of this initiative is to improve the overall quality of life of children, decrease child morality, morbidity and out of pocket expenditure of the poor family. Child Health Screening and early intervention services envisage to cover 30 identified health conditions for early detection, free treatment and management through dedicated mobile Health teams at block level in the country. The mobile health teams comprising (Doctors and Paramedics) carry out screening of all the children in the pre-school age (6 weeks to 5 years) enrolled at Anganwadi Centers at least twice a year besides, screening of all children (6–18) studying in Government and Govt. aided Schools whereas, the newborns are being screened for birth defects in health facilities by service providers and 0–6 weeks during the Home visits by ASHAs.

23. **Blood Services:** Increasing advancement in the field of Transfusion Technology has necessitated enforcing strict control over the quality of Blood and its products. 25 Blood Banks including tertiary care hospitals and 30 Blood Storage units are functional in the UT of J&K. Blood Component Separation Units (BCSU) are functional in Govt. Medical College Hospitals of Jammu/ Srinagar and seven more BCSUs are in a process to procure equipment, five for new GMCs and one each in JLNM Hospital, Srinagar and one in Govt. Hospital, Gandhi Nagar, Jammu. To ensure prevention of transfusion-transmitted infections (TTIs), advanced type of testing is being done in GMC Jammu/GMC Srinagar, i.e., NAT Nucleic Acid Amplification Test. Two Blood Collection and Transport Vans under the program are used for blood donation camps in rural areas; one is under the administrative control of Directorate of Health Services, Jammu and another is under the administrative control of Principal GMC, Srinagar.

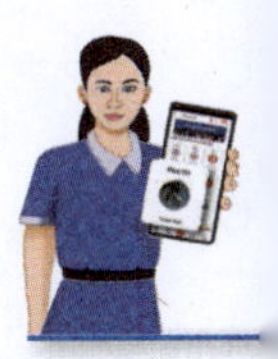

A good laugh and a long sleep are the best cures in the doctor's book.

—Irish Proverb

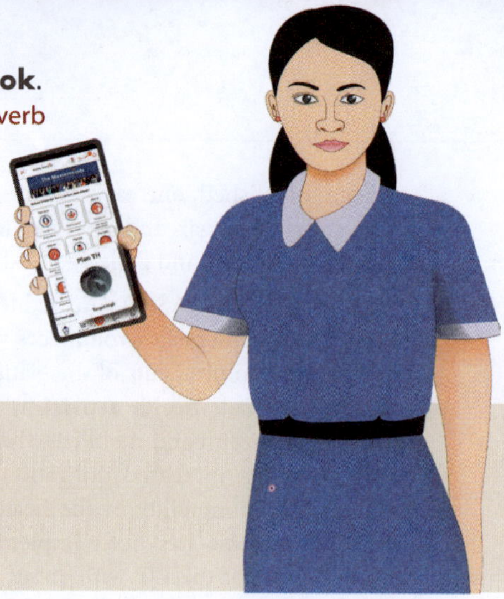

CHAPTER 2

GENERAL ENGLISH AND COMPREHENSION

This Chapter Contains:

- Parts of Speech
- Articles
- Tenses
- Jumbled Words
- Antonyms
- Synonyms
- Idioms and Phrases

PARTS OF SPEECH

The parts of speech play a crucial role in English grammar and composition. They clarify the functions and meaning along with their grammatical use in a sentence. One single word can be used as more than one part of speech in different circumstances. Understanding parts of speech is essential for determining the correct definition of a word.

Nouns

A noun refers to the name of a person, place, thing or object. Basically, anything that names a "thing" is a noun, whether you're talking about a basketball court, San Francisco, Cleopatra or self-preservation.

Nouns are of various types: Common nouns, proper nouns, abstract nouns and concrete nouns; or nouns could be of countable and non-countable types as well.

Pronouns

Pronouns are the substitutes for specific nouns when the reader or listener already knows which specific noun you are referring to.

You might say, "Jenny was supposed to be here at eight," then follow it with "She's always late; next time I'll tell her to be here half an hour earlier."

Instead of saying Jenny's name three times in a row, you substituted *she* and *her,* and your sentences remained grammatically correct.

Adjectives

Adjectives are the words that describe nouns. Think about your favorite movie. How would you describe it to a friend who's never seen it?

You might say the movie was funny, engaging, well-written, or suspenseful. When you're describing the movie with these words, you're using adjectives. An adjective can go right before the noun it's describing ("I have a black dog"), but it doesn't have to. Sometimes, adjectives are at the end of a sentence ("My dog is black").

Verbs

Go! Be amazing! **Run** as fast as you can! **Win** the race! **Congratulate** every participant who **put** in the work and **competed!**

Those bold words are verbs. Verbs are words that describe specific actions, like **running, winning**, and **being** amazing.

Not all verbs refer to literal actions, though. Verbs that refer to feelings or states of being, like **to love** and **to be**, are known as **nonaction verbs**. Conversely, the verbs that do refer to literal actions are known as **action verbs.**

Adverbs

An adverb is a word that describes an adjective, a verb, or another adverb.

I entered the room quietly.

Quietly is describing how you entered (verb) the room.

A cheetah is always faster than a lion.

Always is describing how frequently a cheetah is faster (adjective) than a lion.

Prepositions

Prepositions tell you the relationships between other words in a sentence.

You might say, "I left my bike leaning **against** the garage." In this sentence, **against** is the preposition because it tells us where you left your bike.

Here's another example: "She put the pizza **in** the oven." Without the preposition **in**, we don't know where the pizza is.

Which Preposition to Use and When

Sometimes it may be a little difficult to decide which preposition to use. Thus, the following prepositions need careful handling:

1. **In, at:** 'In' is used with the name of continents, countries, states, sizeable territories and large cities. 'At' is used with towns, villages, etc.
   He is not at home. He lives at Batala.
   He lives in Punjab.
   He lives at Chandarnagar in Bengal.
   But when we speak of very large places, we usually say:
   He lives in London in England (not at London).
   He died in Paris in France. (not at Paris)

2. **At/on:** Compare the following sentences:
   He sat at the table.
   He sat on the table.
   'At' in the first sentence means that he sat with his chair drawn up to the table.
   'On' in the second sentence means that he sat on top of the table.
3. **Between, among:** 'Between' is used in speaking when two persons or things are connected.
   'Among' is used in speaking when more than two persons or things are connected.
   The cat sat between Mohan and Rohan.
   USAGE: 'Between' can also relate to more than two persons or things, when we have a definite number in mind.
4. **In, within:** 'In' means at the end of, 'within' means before the end of.
   He will return in a week. (at the end of week)
   He will return within a week. (before the end of a week)
5. **At, about:** 'At' is used with a fixed moment; 'about' indicates proximity to a certain time.
   He left work at four o'clock.
   It is about four now.
   Expressions like at about four o'clock, at about the time he left work, are therefore wrong.
6. **Till, by:** 'Till' means not earlier than; 'by' means not later than. For example, I was kept waiting till 3 o'clock (up to 3 o'clock). or I shall return home by 3 o'clock (not later than 3 o'clock)
7. **Since, for:** 'Since' as a preposition is used before a noun or phrase denoting some point of time; 'for' is used to donate a period of time; for example, he has been working since morning.
   I have been doing nothing for two hours.
   I have been living in Mumbai since 1980.
   Note: Since is preceded by a verb in perfect tense.
8. **To, till/until-till:** means up to:
   These are used with 'from'. 'To' cannot be used without 'from' though 'however' can be used alone.
   We work from 8 am to 4 pm.
   We work till 4 pm.
   'Until' cannot be used with a negative verb.

Conjunctions

Conjunctions make it possible to build complex sentences that express multiple ideas.

"I like tomato sauce. I like chilli sauce. I don't like mango sauce." Each of these three sentences expresses a clear idea. There's nothing wrong with listing your preferences like this, but it's not the most efficient way to do it.

Consider instead: "I like tomato sauce **and** chilli sauce, **but** I don't like mango sauce.

In this sentence, *and* and *but* are the two conjunctions that link your ideas together.

Interjections

Interjections are a part of speech used to convey or express sudden feelings and emotions. There are no particular rules as to where interjections should be placed in a sentence, but most often, they are seen to appear in the beginning of a sentence. They are used to form exclamatory sentences.

Examples

Here are some examples of interjections to show you how they can be used in sentences effectively.

- **Hurray!** We won the match.
- **Ouch!** That really hurt badly.

ARTICLES

A man. **The** Golden Temple. **An** honest businessman.

The bold words shown above are known as articles. Articles come in two forms: **definite articles** and **indefinite articles**. The definite article, **the** describes one specific noun. **A** and **An** are indefinite articles.

*Did you buy **the** car?*

From the given sentence, we understand that the speaker is referring to a specific car, not any general car.

Now, discuss an indefinite article:

*Did you drive **a** vehicle?*

The given sentence refers to any vehicle which you drove, not any specific vehicle. This shows the use of an indefinite article, i.e., 'a'.

'A' is used with the words which are pronounced with initial consonant sound. E.g., a union, a one-legged man, a pet, a door. **'An'** is used with the words which are pronounced with initial vowel sound. E.g., an apple, an elbow.

TENSES

Tenses refer to the use of different forms of the verbs according to the time of that action.

Tense	Present	Past	Future
Simple	S + V1 + O (Truth/Habit) E.g., He goes for a walk daily.	S + V2 + O (Completed action) E.g., I graduated in 2016.	S + will/shall +V1 + O (Any future action) E.g., I will study French next year.
Continuous	S + is/am/are + V1 + ing + O (Ongoing action) E.g., I am going.	S + was/were + V1 + ing + O (Incomplete task of past) E.g., I was sleeping when he called.	S + will be/ shall be + V1 + ing + O (Future incomplete action) E.g., I will be dancing tomorrow.
Perfect	S + has/ have + V3 + O (Perfectly complete) E.g., I have completed my work.	S + had + V3 + O (Completed action w.r.t. another) E.g., I had left the city.	S + will have + V3 + O (Completed action of future w.r.t. another) E.g., I will have gone by that time.

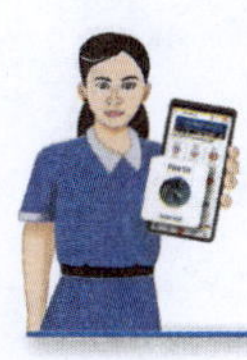

Contd...

Tense	Present	Past	Future
Perfect Continuous	S + has/have + been + V1 + ing + O (Started in past and Still continue) E.g., I have been writing since 1 pm	S + had been + V1 + ing + O (Past incomplete action w.r.t. another) E.g., I had been living in Mumbai for three years.	S + will have been + V1 +ing + O (Future incomplete action w.r.t. another) E.g., She will have been reading a novel.

JUMBLED WORDS

Read the following words and arrange them to make a meaningful sentence:

1. dealer / favor / that/ was / in / of /that proposal / said / he/ the
   Dealer said that he was in the favor of that proposal.
2. was / performance /impressed /with/ very / his/he
   He was very impressed with his performance.

ANTONYMS

A word opposite in meaning or sense to a given word is called its antonym. Antonyms are of three types:

1. **Words without any prefix or suffix. Such words are called direct Antonyms.**
   Study the following examples:

Words	Antonyms
Abundance	Dearth
Abject	Elevated
Zenith	Nadir

2. **Antonyms can be formed by using a prefix before a word.**
   Some important prefixes are: In, un, dis. Mark the following examples:

Words	Antonyms
Ability	Inability
Well	Unwell
Advantage	Disadvantage

3. **Some Antonyms can be formed by changing the suffix of a given word.** Mark the following examples:

Words	Antonyms
Careful	Careless
Faithful	Faithless
Advantage	Disadvantage

SYNONYMS

A synonym is a word that has almost the same meaning as another word. For example, a synonym for beautiful is stunning.

- She is a beautiful girl.
- She is a stunning girl.

In this part, antonyms and synonyms of real importance have been given.

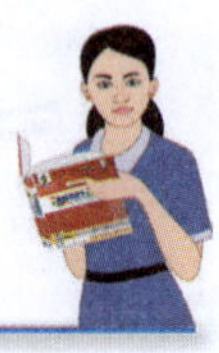

Word	Antonym	Synonym
Abandon	Retain	Leave
Absurd	Relevant	Illogical
Alive	Dead	Lively, Vivacious
Abundance	Scarcity	Plenty
Assemble	Disperse	Gather
Audible	Inaudible	Detectable, Observable
Blunt	Sharp	Unsharpened, Edgeless
Blessing	Curse	Grace, Benediction
Bold	Timid	Courageous
Benediction	Malediction	Blessing
Care	Neglect	Concern
Coarse	Fine	Crude, Unrefined
Contract	Expand	Shrink
Concord	Discord	Harmony
Conceal	Reveal	Obscure, Camouflage
Dense	Sparse	Opaque, Solid, Close-knit
Despair	Hope	Despondency, Dejection
Emigrant	Immigrant	Alien, Foreigner
Firm	Shaky	Condensed, Solid
Foreign	Native	Non-native, Overseas, Distant
Fresh	Stale	Revived, Lively
Futile	Fruitful	Inefficacious
Inferior	Superior	Subservient, Junior
Ignorance	Knowledge	Incomprehension
Gather	Scatter	Congregate
Giant	Dwarf	Gigantic, Colossal
Grieve	Rejoice	Mourn, Lament
Harmony	Discord	Euphony
Optional	Compulsory	Discretional
Optimist	Pessimist	Idealizer, Propitious
Obligatory	Optional	Statutory
Pardon	Punish	Condonation
Praise	Condemn/blame	Commend
Poison	Antidote	Toxin
Plenty	Scarcity	Plethora
Predecessor	Successor	Precursor, Prototype
Peculiar	Normal	Idiosyncratic
Ruthless	Merciful	Cold-blooded
Respect	Insult	Adoration
Steady	Unstable	Unwavering

Contd...

Word	Antonym	Synonym
Severe	Mild	Grievous
Scold	Praise	Rebuke
Theory	Practical	Hypothesis, Dogma
Vacant	Occupied	Deserted, Uninhabited

IDIOMS AND PHRASES

Idiom is a phrase whose meaning is different from the literal meaning of the given words, we have to figure out its hidden meaning. They are commonly used in English language and common vocabulary.

Some of the idioms and phrases of clinical importance are given below:

- **Green around the gills:** Looking sick; e.g., Due to this changing weather, my child is looking green around the gills.
- **Feel on the top of the world**: Feeling healthy; e.g., Tashir has been feeling on the top of the world ever since she has cleared NORCET exam.
- **Nothing but skin and bones:** Be very thin; e.g., I hardly recognized my childhood friend because he is nothing but skin and bones now.
- **On the mend:** Healing; e.g., Her leg mended slowly after surgery.
- **Picture of health:** Ideal example of health; e.g., Narendra Modi is a picture of health these days.
- **Out of condition/shape**: Not in a good physical health; e.g., My trekking trip made me realize that I'm out of condition now and need to work on it.
- **Foot-in-mouth disease:** Habit of unintentionally saying foolish things; e.g., He has foot-in-mouth disease when asked to give a speech.
- **Get a black eye**: Get a dark eye after being hit over that area; e.g., The thief ran away after giving me a black eye.
- **Black and blue:** Bruised/beaten badly; e.g., He was beaten black and blue.
- **Fill a prescription**: Get medicines from pharmacy as ordered by doctor; e.g., One should always fill a prescription in order to heal quickly.
- **Bundle of nerves:** A very nervous person; e.g., After any frightening experience, anyone can be a bundle of nerves.
- **Catch one's death of cold:** Become very ill; e.g., During winters, going out with wet hair can make you catch one's death of cold.
- **A dose of one's own medicine**: The same treatment that one gives to others; e.g., Dr Neha gave a dose of one's own medicine to everyone in the office during the emergence of conjunctivitis.
- **Breath one's last:** To die; e.g., He breathed his last with his loved ones.
- **Roll up your sleeves:** Get ready; e.g., Please roll up your sleeve as nurse will be injecting your dose of medicine.
- **At death's door:** Near death; e.g., My grandfather was so ill that he was at death's door for three days.
- **As fit as a fiddle/In the pink of health/Alive and kicking:** Be healthy and physically fit; e.g., Despite being 94 years of age, my grandmother is as fit as a fiddle.
- **Back on one's feet:** Physically healthy again; e.g., He was suffering from a critical disease but his doctor made him back on his feet again.
- **Snake oil:** Medicine of unproven value; e.g., These days there are a lot of snake oil salesmen.
- **Clean Bill of Health:** A report that someone is healthy; e.g., After annual health check, my mother was given a clean bill of health by the doctors.
- **A bitter pill to swallow:** An unpleasant fact that one must accept; e.g., Our people have swallowed a bitter pill during the Independence struggle.
- **Flare up:** Sudden outburst, e.g., Corona outbreak flared up in 2021 as well.
- **Go under the knife:** Have any surgery; e.g., My dog needs to go under the knife to survive.
- **Splitting headache:** A severe headache; e.g., Hectic health care jobs can give splitting headache at times.
- **As pale as a ghost:** Extremely pale; e.g., Due to iron deficiency, my father became as pale as a ghost.

PRACTICE QUESTIONS

1. Fill in the blanks with appropriate prepositions.
at, in, on, by, to, with, of, after, into, about, from

i. The two brothers met __________a long time.
ii. She asked me_________my business.
iii. I am coming ___________ the railway station.

2. Fill in the blanks with appropriate prepositions.
along, against, for, above, with, in, before, across, between, of

i. How many boys in the class weigh_________sixty pounds?
ii. His school is situated__________ the road.
iii. Finish this work __________ sunset.

3. Each occupation has its own ....; bankers, lawyers and computer professionals, for example, all use different languages which outsiders have difficulty in following.

a. Merits b. Disadvantages
c. Rewards d. Jargon

4. Biological clocks are of such .... adaptive value to living organisms that we would expect most organisms to .... them.

a. Clear – avoid b. Meager – evolve
c. Significant – eschew d. Obvious – possess

5. Many people at that time believed that spices help preserve food; however, Hall found that many marketed spices were .... bacteria, molds and yeasts.

a. Devoid of b. Teeming with
c. Improved by d. Destroyed by

6. Which of the following is an antonym of 'Docile'?

a. Unmanageable b. Dutiful
c. Submissive d. Painful

7. Which of the following is an antonym of 'Erudite'?

a. Professional b. Stately
c. Short d. Ignorant

8. Which of the following is a synonym of CONCILIATORY?

a. Foolish b. Soothing
c. Advisory d. Over proud

9. Which of the following is a synonym of OBDURATE?

a. Shaky b. Stubborn
c. Hostile d. Boring

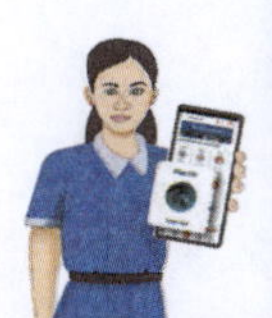

10. Arrange the given sentences to form a meaningful paragraph.

A. The two neighbors never fought each other.

B. Fights involving three male fiddler crabs have been recorded, but the status of the participants was unknown.

C. They pushed or grappled only with the intruder.

D. We recorded 17 cases in which a resident who was fighting an intruder was joined by an immediate neighbor, an ally.

E. We, therefore, tracked 268 intruder males until we saw them fighting a resident male.

The proper sequence should be:

a. BEDAC b. DEBAC
c. BDCAE d. BCEDA

11. Arrange the following to form a meaningful sentence. He said

A. Here is the cat
B. Throughout the night
C. Which had been playing havoc with things
D. That ate the rat

The proper sequence should be:

a. ADBC b. ADCB
c. BACD d. BCAD

12. Read the following sentences and select the correct words from the pair to complete them:

i. I am ________ of my success. (confidant, confident)
ii. No ________ explanation on this issue please! (farther, further)
iii. Is there ________ in the hall? (anyone, none)
iv. The father ________ the son to stop fighting. (advised, adviced)
v. Mona exclaimed she is enjoying wearing her ________ dress. (latest, later)

13. Fill the suitable articles in the blanks:

i. Fred is ________ honest man.
ii. Ashoka was ________ just king.
iii. Lion allowed ________ mouse to leave.
iv. You have fixed ________ appointment with ________ physician.
v. Will Roma take ________ picture of us?

14. Fill the sentence with correct word:
The constable is ________ the station.

a. At b. On
c. Over d. Under

15. Fill the sentence with correct word:
The moon will not rise ________ 6 o'clock.

a. Before b. Since
c. Till d. After

16. Choose the option with grammatical error in the following sentence:
I visit/Niagara Falls/last weekend.

a. I visit b. Niagara Falls
c. last weekend d. No error

17. Choose the option with grammatical error in the following sentence:
The man which works here is from Britain.

a. The man
b. Which works
c. Here is
d. From Britain

18. Choose the option with grammatical error in the following sentence:
She's married with a dentist.

a. She's married b. With a
c. Dentist d. No error

19. Select the correct meaning of the underlined idiom used in the given sentence:
The medical authorities took him to task for his negligence.

a. Punished him b. Provided extra tasks
c. Asked him to resign d. Criticized him

20. Select the correct meaning of the underlined idiom:
The Adani group once reached on its last legs.

a. About to perish
b. About to be lucrative
c. About to boom
d. All of the above

ANSWER KEY

Exercise Questions

1.	i. after, ii. about, iii. from	2.	i. above, ii. across. iii. Before	3.	d	4.	d	5.	b
6.	a	7.	d	8.	b	9.	b	10.	a
11.	b	12.	i. confident ii. further iii. anyone iv. advised v. latest	13.	i. an ii. a iii. the iv. an, the v. a			14.	a
15.	a	16.	a	17.	b			18.	b
19.	d	20.	a						

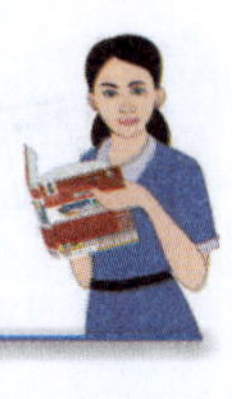

"One day in perfect health is much."

—Arabic proverb

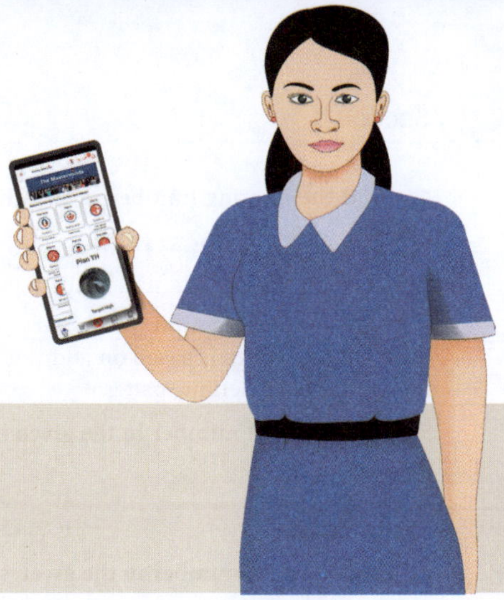

CHAPTER 3

GENERAL INTELLIGENCE AND REASONING ABILITY

CODING-DECODING

Alphabet test-based questions are generally asked which require an understanding of positions of alphabets in the series.

Forward number	Alphabet	Forward number	Alphabet
1	A	14	N
2	B	15	O
3	C	16	P
4	D	17	Q
5	E	18	R
6	F	19	S
7	G	20	T
8	H	21	U
9	I	22	V
10	J	23	W
11	K	24	X
12	L	25	Y
13	M	26	Z

1. **In a certain code language, "BOY" is written as "21225". What will be the code for "GIRL" in the same language?**
   a. 791218 b. 792181
   c. 791812 d. 791281
2. **In a certain code language, "You are good." is written as "la ba ma" and "I am bad." is written as "ca sa pa". What will be the code for "Am I good?" in the same language?**
   a. sa ca ma b. sa la ma
   c. sa ca ba d. sa pa ca
3. **In a certain code, "APPLE" is written as "ZOOKD". What will be the code for "BANANA" in the same language?**
   a. AAMZMZ b. AZMZNZ
   c. AZMZBZ d. AZMZMZ
4. **How many letters are there between 8th letter from left and 7th letter from right in alphabet series?**
   a. 11 b. 7
   c. 8 d. 10
5. **In a certain code, FILE is written as 7465 and IDEAL is written as 43586. How will DEAF be written in that code language?**
   a. 3587 b. 3467
   c. 3764 d. 3827

ANALOGY

Analogy means similarity, i.e., a particular relationship between words/letters/numbers will be given and another similar relationship we have to find from the options.

Questions:

1. **"Cock" is related to "Hen" in the same way as "Peacock" is related to:**
   a. Peahen b. Parrot
   c. Pigeon d. Bird
2. **Brick: Wall: House**
   a. Eyes: Lashes: See b. Water: River: Sea
   c. Hands: Legs: Body d. Cell: Tissue: Organ
3. **12 : 144 : : 17 :**
   a. 199 b. 289
   c. 241 d. 179
4. **ASTN : ZTSO : : MSUB :**
   a. ALCY b. LTTC
   c. LRRC d. LTTA
5. **BOY : 6 : : HONEY :**
   a. 8 b. 6
   c. 4 d. 7

NUMBER SYSTEM

Number series is a sequential arrangement of numbers in which numbers follow a certain pattern. This pattern can be based on:

i. **Addition/Subtraction of numbers:** If the number series in increasing slowly, then it will be addition series otherwise if the numbers are decreasing slowly, then that will be a subtraction series.

1. **Find the next number in the given series: 7, 12, 19, 28, 39, …**
   a. 51 b. 52
   c. 53 d. 54
2. **Find the next number in the given series: 40, 30, 22, 16, ……**
   a. 12b. 16
   c. 14d. 50

ii. **Multiplication/Division of numbers:** If the number series in increasing rapidly, then it will be multiplication series otherwise if the numbers are decreasing rapidly, then that will be a division series.

3. **Find the next number in the given series: 20, 100, 600, 4200, 33600, …..**
   a. 302300 b. 302400
   c. 302600 d. 302700

4. **Find the missing number in the given series: 648, 216, 108, 36, ..., 6.**
   a. 16   b. 24
   c. 18   d. 12

iii. **Addition/Subtraction of Squares/Cubes of numbers:** At times, the series is based on addition or subtraction of squares or cubes of a definite pattern.

5. **Find the next number in the given series: 212, 208, 199, 183, ...**
   a. 158   b. 153
   c. 143   d. 130

6. **Find the next number in the given series: 8, 27, 64, 125, ...**
   a. 224   b. 326
   c. 260   d. 216

BLOOD RELATIONS

Blood relations are the relations between two or more persons. It can be maternal relations which are relations on mother's side. It can be paternal relations which are on father's side.

Trick: To solve such questions easily, you should make a diagram by adding various symbols.

Sl. No.	Individual/Relation	Symbol
1.	Man	+
2.	Woman	-
3.	Husband-Wife	+ < > -
4.	Brother-Sister	+ -
5.	Brother-Brother	+ +
6.	Sister-Sister	- -

1. **Example: A is the father of B, C is the brother of A, F is the sister of B. If M is the father of A, then establish relationship between F and C.**
   a. Husband and Wife   b. Daughter and Father
   c. Grandmother and Granddaughter
   d. Niece and Uncle

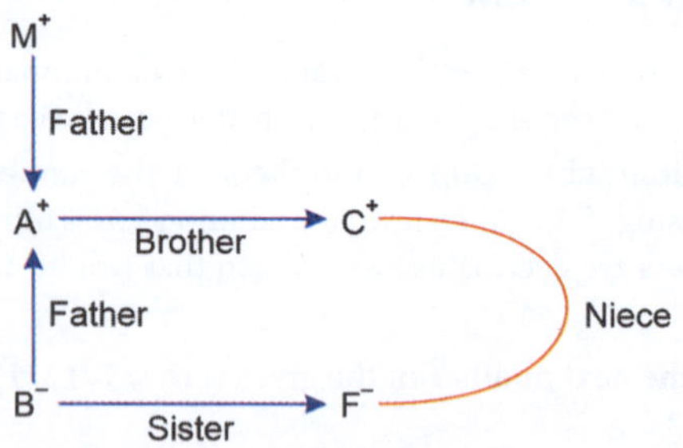

2. **By showing a picture of a boy Manish said, "He is the son of the only son of my mother." How is Manish related to that boy?**
   a. Brother   b. Cousin
   c. Father   d. Uncle

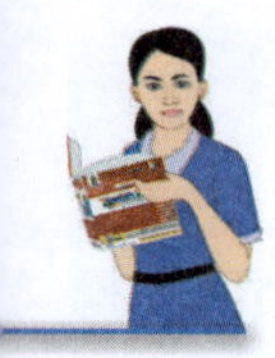

3. **If L@M means L is the wife of M, L#M means L is the son of M, L5M means L is the sister of M, L$M means L is the father of M. Which of the following expressions shows Y as the brother of Z?**
   a. Z#X$Y   b. Z%X$Y
   c. Z%Y$X   d. Y%Z$X

DIRECTION SENSE TEST

Direction sense test is a test based on the movement of a person or object in different directions and then finally deciding the direction with respect to another object given in the situation. This can be done by understanding the eight directions which are North, South, East, West, North-East, North-West, South-East and South-West.

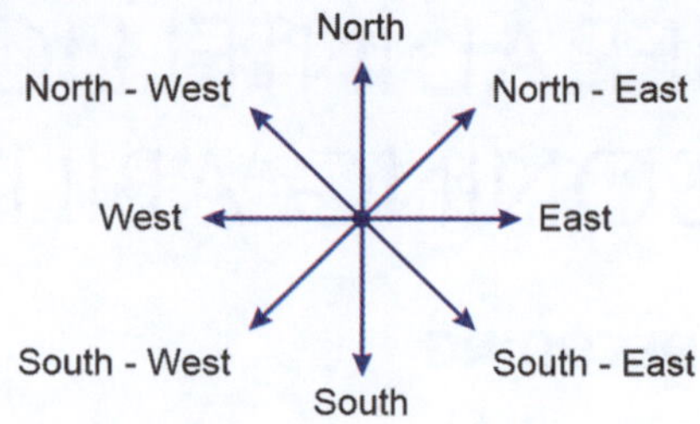

Figure: Eight directions

1. **A clock is showing wrong time such that at 2:00 am the hour hand points toward North West.In which direction does the hour hand point at 6:00 am?**
   a. North-West   b. North-East
   c. West   d. South-East

2. **Delhi is to the West of Noida. Gurugram is to the South of Delhi. Faridabad is to the East of Gurugram. Then Faridabad is toward which direction of Delhi?**
   a. North   b. South-West
   c. South-East   d. South

3. **Reema walked 30 m toward the North. Then she turned right and walked 45 m. Then she turned right and walks 45 m. Then she turned left and walks 5 m. Finally, she turned left and walked 15 m. How many meters away she is now from the starting position?**
   a. 25 m   b. 50 m
   c. 40 m   d. 65 m

SITTING ARRANGEMENT

Sitting arrangement is a pattern followed by objects/persons who are sitting in any row or a circle. One has to determine the position of all with respect to each other.

Note: When direction of persons/objects in a row is not specified, by default we assume that they are facing North.

Directions (Q 1 to 3): Eight friends, namely, K, A, B, P, T, Y, V and D are sitting around a circular table and each of them is facing the center:

I. K is second to the right of T who is the neighbor of B and V
II. P is not the neighbor of K
III. V is the neighbor of Y
IV. A is not between P and D
V. D is not between Y and P
VI. D is not an immediate neighbor of K

1. **Who is sitting exactly opposite to A?**
   a. K   b. V
   c. B   d. T

2. **How many people sit between D and V?**
   a. Two   b. One
   c. Three   d. Five

3. **Who sits third to the right of Y?**
   a. T   b. B
   c. A   d. D

MIRROR AND WATER IMAGE

The reflection of any object in mirror is known as a Mirror image and reflection of any object in water is known as a Water image.
In mirror image, there are two cases. One is when mirror is placed vertically. Then the LHS and RHS of image get interchanged. In another case, mirror is placed horizontally, where top and bottom of the image get interchanged.

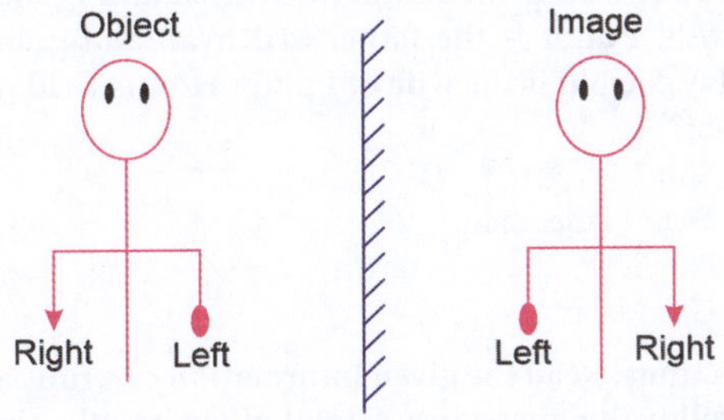

Figure i. Mirror placed vertically, where LHS and RHS are interchanged

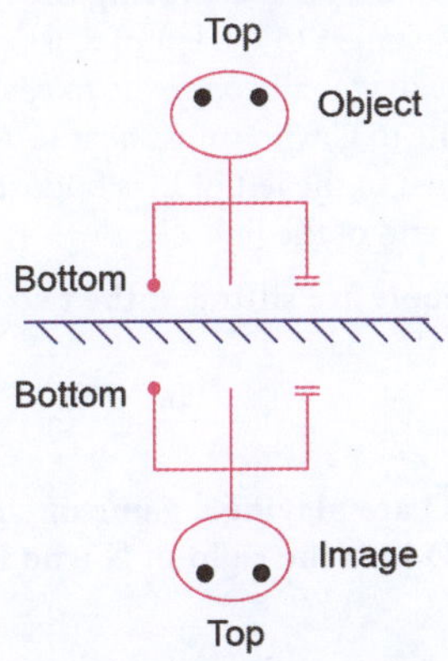

Figure ii. Mirror placed horizontally, where Top and Bottom are interchanged

1. **If the mirror is placed vertically, then identify the correct mirror image of O B S T I N A T E?**
   a. ƎTAИIT2ᙠO   b. BOSTINATE
   c. ETANITSBO   d. SOBTNIATE

2. **If an object is placed on the front of the mirror as shown in the image, what will be its mirror image?**

a. 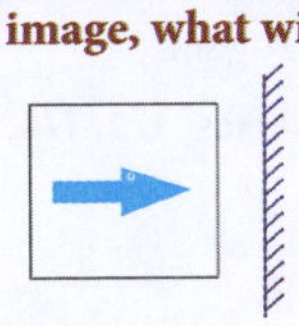
b. 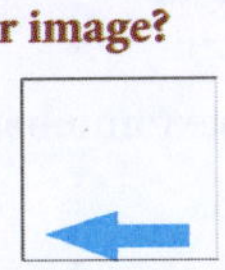
c. 
d. 

Water image is formed when any object is placed near any water source, for example any pond, river or sea. In this case, the image gets inverted.

Note: It is same like the mirror image, when mirror is placed horizontally.

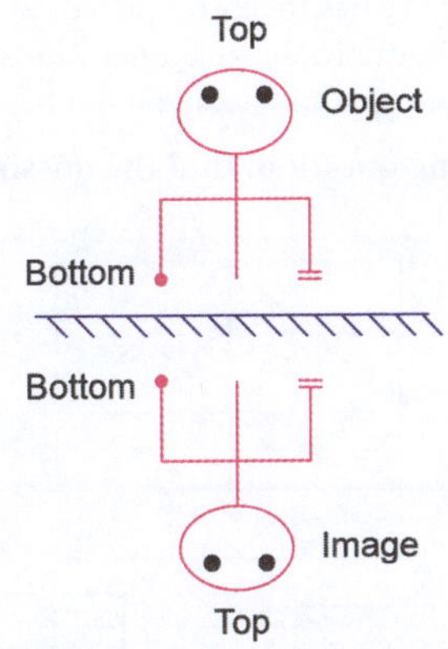

Figure: Objected inverted in case of water image

3. **Which one of the following is the water image of E 8 t 4 e 9 C?**

E 8 T 4 e 9 C
   a. Ǝ8ʇ4ɘ9Ɔ   b. E8ʇ4ɘ9Ɔ
   c. E8ɫ↋ɘ6C   d. E8ɫ↋ɘ6C

4. **Choose the water image of the following figure:**

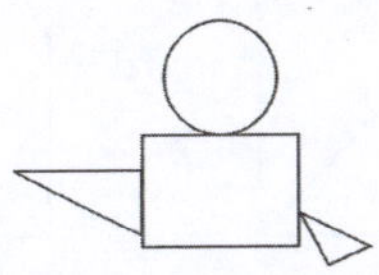

a. 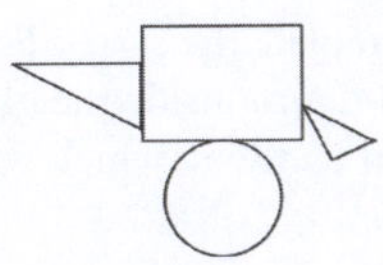
b. 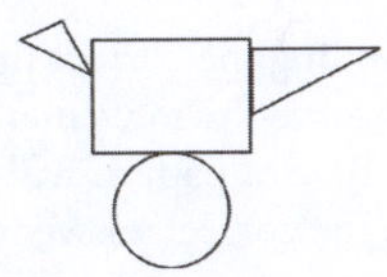
c. 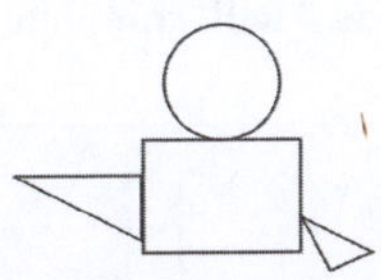
d. 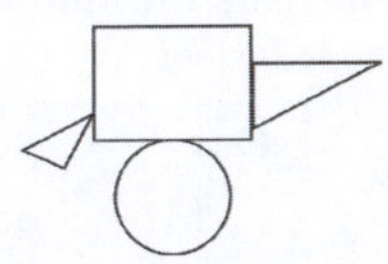

FIGURE-BASED QUESTIONS

Figure-based questions are based on different orientation of any figure. Following are the few types:

i. When question figure is present in the given options and we have to find it out:

1. **Find the option in which the given figure is embedded.**

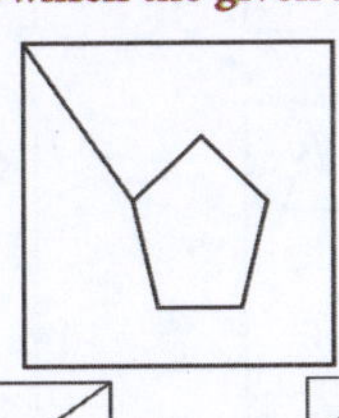

a. 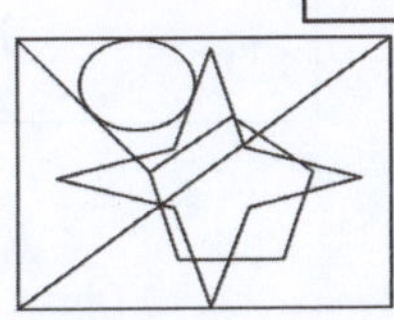
b. 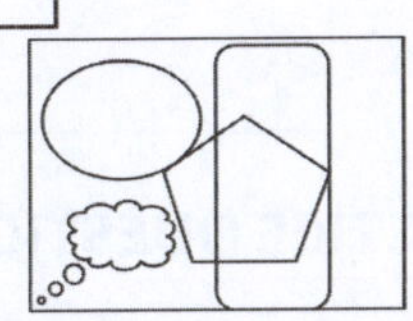
c. 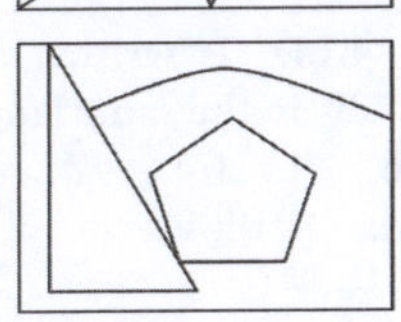
d. 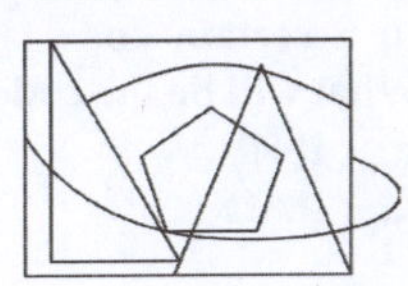

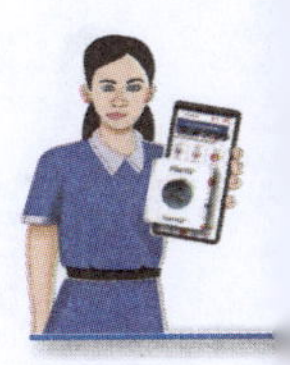

ii. When given figure has to be completed, we need to observe the pattern of the figure in the given questions. (Mirror image and water image concepts can help you out here.)

2. In the following question, find the missing part of the given figure.

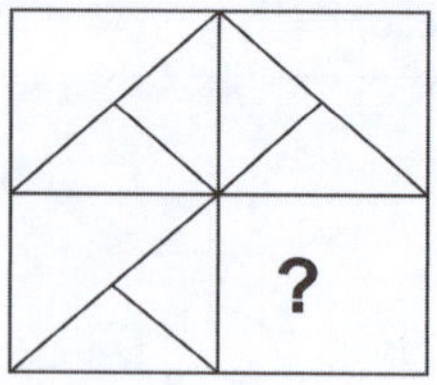

a. 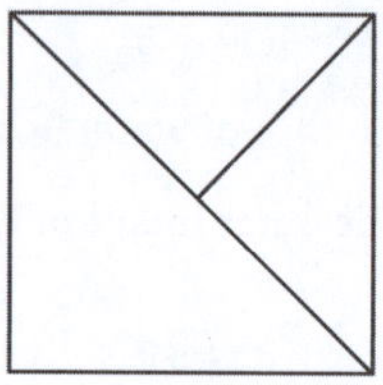
b. 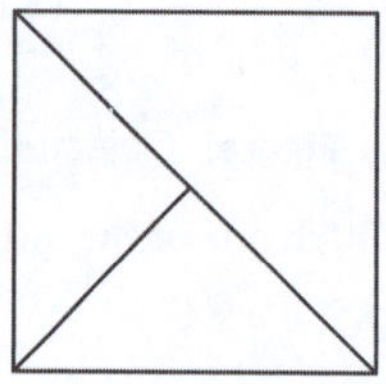

c. 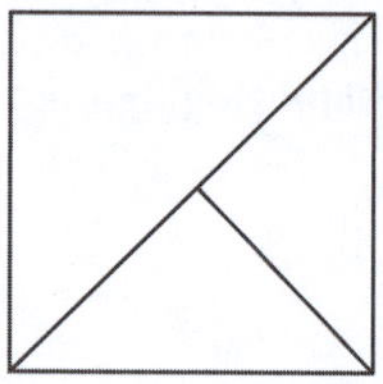
d. 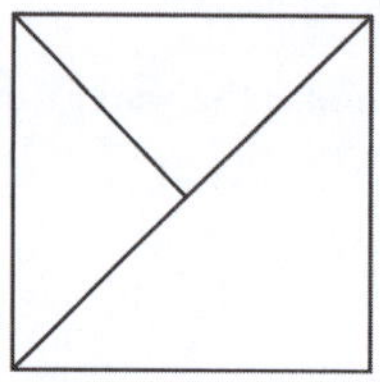

iii. Finding the correct figure to complete the series. For this type, observe the movement to small figure inside the given square. A type of pattern will be formed by them, which will direct us to the correct answer.

3. Which of the following options will complete the given figure series?

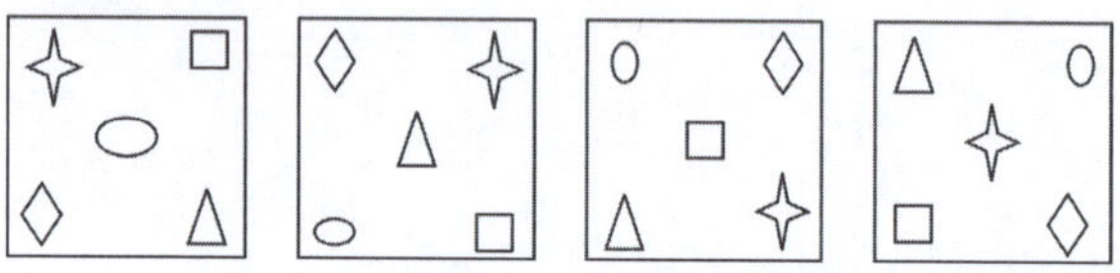

a. 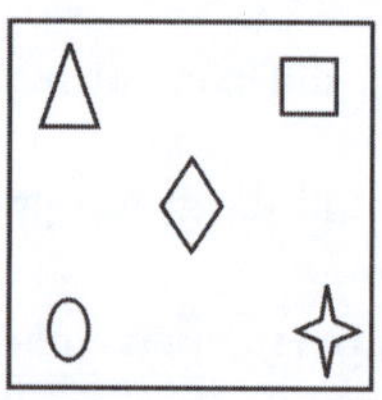
b. 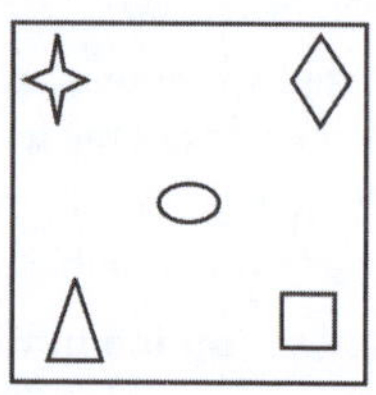

c. 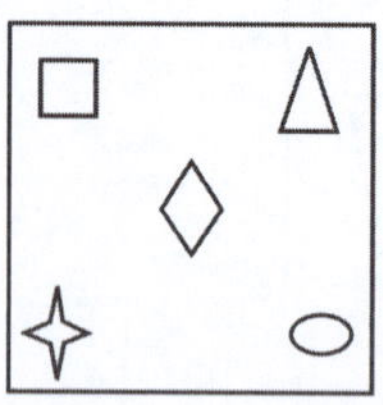
d. 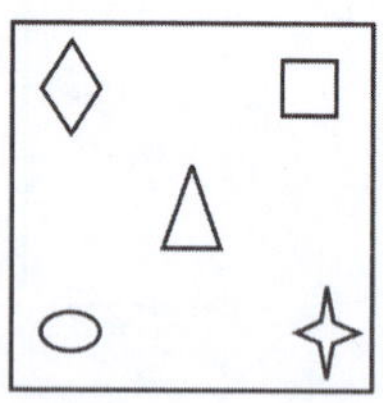

PRACTICE QUESTIONS

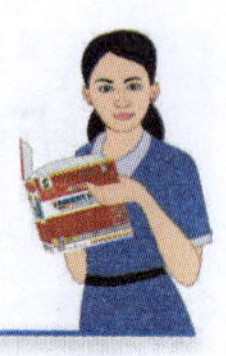

1. In a certain code language, "BED" is written as "YVW". What will be the code for "ROSE" in the same language?

a. ILHV b. ILVH
c. ILMN d. VHLM

2. In a certain code language, "KITE" is written as "LHUF". What will be the code for "THREAD" in the same language?

a. UISFBE b. UISFEB
c. UIFSEB d. UIFBE

3. Complete the given series: 10, 11, 12, 15, 13, 14, ...

a. 14 b. 15
c. 13 d. 11

4. Complete the given series: 7, 12, 16, 19, 28, 39, ...

a. 7 b. 12
c. 16 d. 19

5. Kriday is a son of Santosh's father's sister. Pankaj is the son of Surbhi who is the mother of Girish and grandmother of Santosh. Pulkit is the father of Khyati and grandfather of Kriday. Surbhi is the wife of Pulkit. How is Kriday related to Surbhi?

a. Son
b. Data inadequate
c. Nephew
d. Grandson

6. Directions: Read the given information carefully and answer the following questions: A total of ten people, five men and five women are sitting in two parallel lines, facing each other. Five men, P, Q, R, S and T are facing to the South and the five women, A, B, C, D and E are facing the North.

I. Q, who is just next to the left of S, is opposite to E.
II. R and B are diagonally opposite to each other.
III. T is opposite to C who is just next to A.
IV. D, who is just to the left of E, is opposite to S.
V. A is at one end of the line

Which two people are sitting at the two extreme ends of the line?

a. T, Q b. P, R
c. R, S d. S, Q

7. L, M, N, and O are playing a game of chess. L, N, and O, M are partners. O is to the right of N who is facing West. Then M is facing?

a. North b. South
c. East d. West

8. Speedometer is related to Speed as Odometer is to:

a. Speed
b. Direction
c. Distance
d. Car

9. Fox is related to Clever as Kids is to:

a. Beautiful b. Ugly
c. Innocent d. Arrogant

10. Find the next number in the given series: 1/2, 1/4, 1/8, 1/16, ...

a. 1/32 b. 1/64
c. 1/128 d. 1/48

11. Find the next number in the given series: 20, 10, 15, 37.5, ...

a. 125.25 b. 25.25
c. 145.25 d. 131.25

12. Find the correct water image of the word: ADVANCE

a. VDAVИCE b. ƎƆИAVDA
c. ƎƆNⱯΛDⱯ d. ƎƆИAƆVA

13. The given figure is embedded in which of the following options?

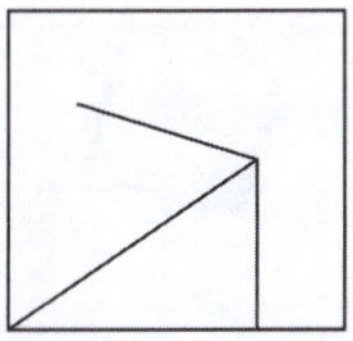

a. 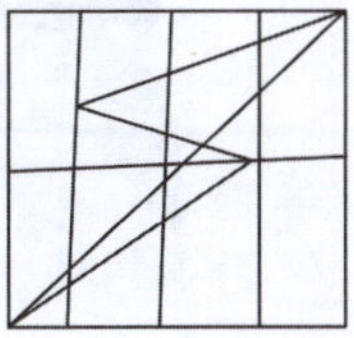 b. 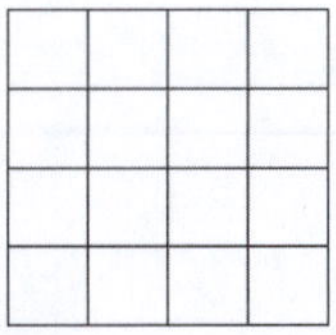

c. 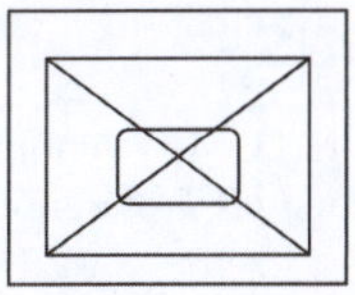 d. 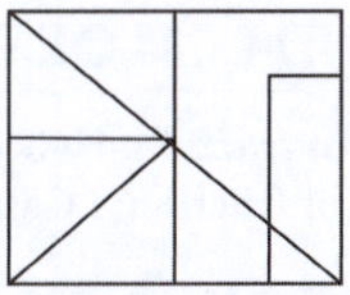

14. Which of the following options completes the series?

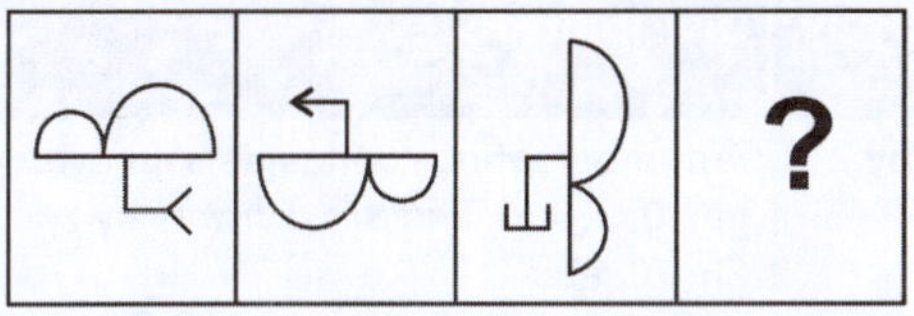

a. 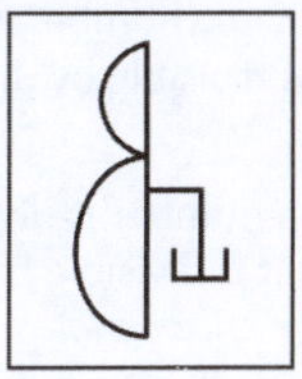 b. 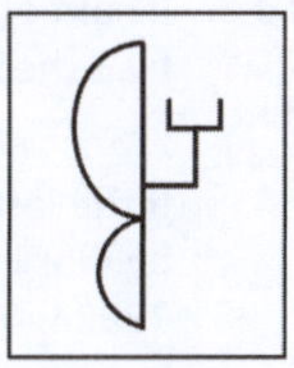

c. 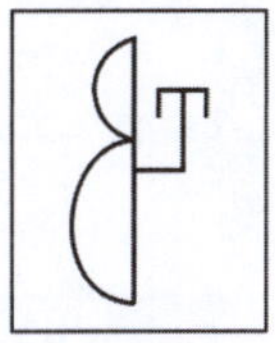 d. 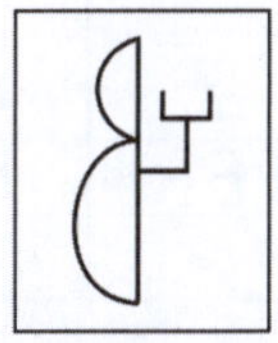

15. Select the correct option to complete the figure:

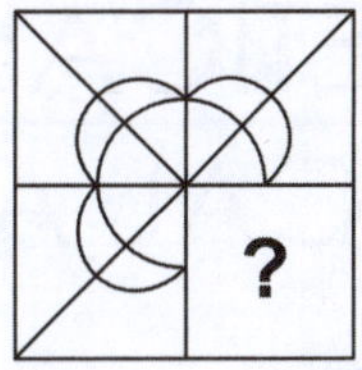

a. 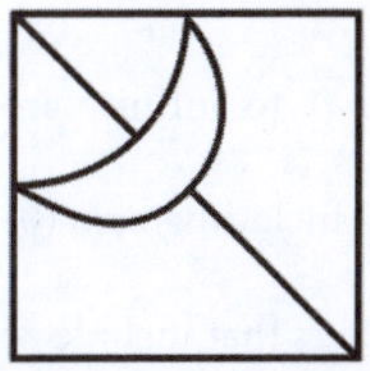 b. 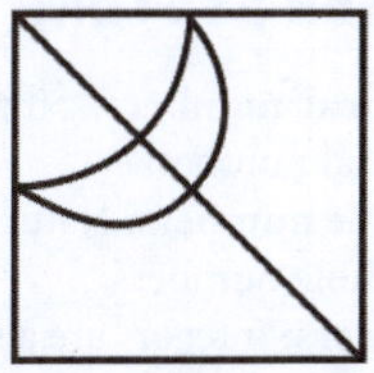

c. 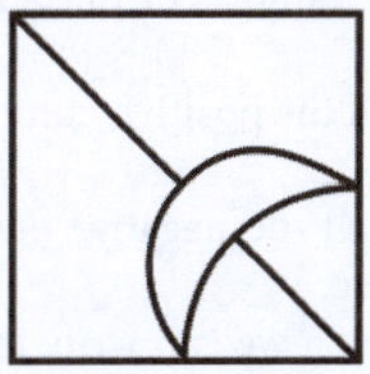 d. 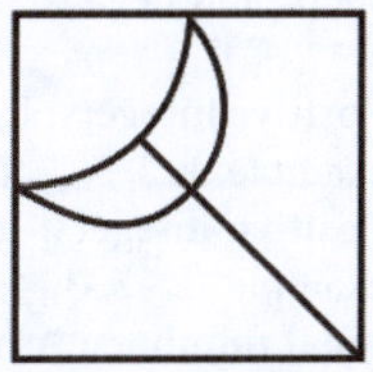

ANSWERS

Coding-Decoding

1.	c	2.	a	3.	d	4.	a	5.	a

Analogy

1.	a	2.	d	3.	b	4.	b	5.	b

Number System

1.	b	2.	a	3.	b	4.	c	5.	a	6.	d

Blood Relations

1.	d	2.	c	3.	c

Direction Sense Test

1.	d	2.	c	3.	b

Sitting Arrangement

1.	b	2.	a	3.	b

Mirror and Water Image

1.	a	2.	d	3.	d	4.	d

Figure-Based Questions

1.	a	2.	b	3.	c

Exercise Questions

1.	a	2.	a	3.	b
4.	c	5.	d	6	b
7.	a	8.	c	9.	c
10.	a	11.	d	12.	a
13.	a	14.	d	15.	b

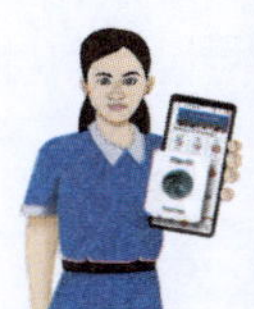

A man's health can be judged by which he takes two at a time - pills or stairs.

—Joan Welsh

CHAPTER 4

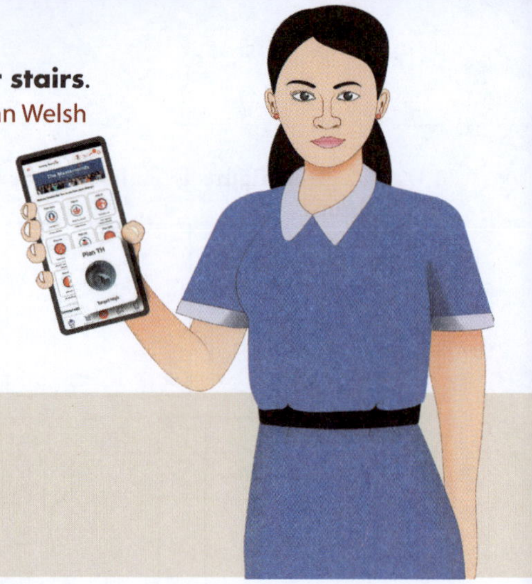

ARITHMETICAL AND NUMERICAL ABILITY

NUMBER SYSTEM

1. **Natural numbers:** Numbers from 1 to infinity are known as natural numbers.
2. **Whole numbers:** Natural numbers including zero (0) are known as whole numbers.
3. **Integers:** Integers are a set of numbers that include zero, positive numbers, and negative numbers. Examples of Integers: – 1, -12, 6, 15.
   - **Positive integers:** It includes all the positive numbers. For
   - example, 1, 2, 3, 4, 5, 6….., etc.
   - **Positive integers:** It includes all the negative numbers. For example -1, -2,-3,-4,-5,-6….., etc.
4. **Rational numbers:** A number which we can write in p/q form, where p is an integer and q is not equal to zero is known as a rational number. For example: 4/5, 6/7, 1/5, etc.
5. **Irrational numbers:** The numbers which cannot be expressed in p/q form are known as irrational numbers. Also, the decimal expressions of these numbers are nonterminating and nonrepeating. For example:, $\sqrt{2}$, $\sqrt{3}$, $\sqrt{5}$….etc.
6. **Real numbers:** The combination of rational and irrational numbers is known as real numbers. For example: 11/23, etc.
7. **Prime numbers:** The number which is divisible by only 1 or by itself is known as prime number. For example: 2, 3, 5, 7, etc.
8. **Composite numbers:** Numbers that have more than two factors are known as composite numbers. For example: 4, 6, 8, etc.
9. **Co-prime numbers:** Numbers having only one common factor are called co-prime numbers. For example: (3,7) (8,9), etc.

LCM AND HCF

- **Least common multiple (LCM):** The least number which is exactly divisible by two or more numbers is known as LCM.
  Example: If we consider the multiples of 16 and 20, we get;
  Multiples of 16 are 16, 32, 48, 64, **80**,…
  Multiples of 20 are 20, 40, 60, **80**,…
  We can see that the first common multiple for both the numbers is 80. So, LCM of 16 and 20 is 80.
- **Highest common factor (HCF):** The greatest factor between two or more numbers is known as HCF.
  Example: Highest common factor of 144, 104, and 160. Now write the prime factors of 144, 104 and 160.

$$144 = 2 \times 2 \times 2 \times 2 \times 3 \times 3$$
$$104 = 2 \times 2 \times 2 \times 13$$
$$160 = 2 \times 2 \times 2 \times 2 \times 2 \times 5$$

  The common factors of 144, 104 and 160 are $2 \times 2 \times 2 = 8$
  Therefore, HCF (144, 104, 160) = 8

HCF AND LCM OF FRACTIONS

- **HCF of fraction:** HCF of numerators/LCM of denominators
- **LCM of fraction:** LCM of numerators/ HCF of denominators

TEST OF DIVISIBILITY

Divisibility by number	Divisibility Rule
Divisible by 2	A number whose unit digit is an even number, i.e., 0, 2, 4, 6, and 8 is divisible by 2, e.g., 78, 86, 70, etc.
Divisible by 3	If sum of all the digits of any number is divisible by 3 then the number is divisible by 3, e.g., 39, 81, etc.
Divisible by 4	If the last two digits of a number is divisible by 4 or include 00 then it is divisible by 4, e.g., 78924, 6732, etc.
Divisible by 5	Numbers whose unit digit is 0 or 5 are divisible by 5, e.g., 780,7895, etc.
Divisible by 6	A number which is divisible by 2 and 3 both is divisible by 6, e.g., 4536, 8124, etc.
Divisible by 8	If the last three digits of a number is divisible by 8 or include 000 then it is divisible by 8, e.g., 5647472.
Divisible by 9	If sum of all the digits of any number is divisible by 9 then the number is divisible by 9, e.g., 3933, 729, etc.
Divisible by 10	Any number whose unit digit is 0 is divisible by 10, e.g., 3930, 7290, etc.
Divisible by 11	If the difference of the sums of the alternative digits of a number is divisible by 11 then the number is divisible by 11, e.g., 1331, **10824**,etc.

Example: Check if the number 2347974 is divisible by 8 or 11?

Solution: For checking any number's divisibility with 8, we check for the divisibility of last three digits of a number by 8 or the presence of 000. So, here, 000 is not there. We will check the divisibility of 974 by 8.

974 is not completely divisible by 8.

For checking any number's divisibility with 11, we check for the difference of sum of alternate digits of the given number. If it comes out to be a factor of 11 then it will be divisible by 11.

So, (2+4+9+4) – (3+7+7) = 19 – 17 = 2

This brings us to the conclusion that the given number is **neither divisible by 8 nor by 11**.

SIMPLIFICATION

BODMAS Rule

The BODMAS rule is essential in many mathematical problems. The full form of BODMAS is:

- B – Brackets,
- O – Order of powers or roots,
- D – Division,
- M – Multiplication,
- A – Addition,
- S – Subtraction.

IMPORTANT ALGEBRAIC FORMULAS

Some important algebraic formulas are as follows:

- $a^2 - b^2 = (a - b)(a + b)$
- $(a + b)^2 = a^2 + 2ab + b^2$
- $a^2 + b^2 = (a + b)^2 - 2ab$
- $(a - b)^2 = a^2 - 2ab + b^2$
- $(a + b + c)^2 = a^2 + b^2 + c^2 + 2ab + 2bc + 2ca$
- $(a - b - c)^2 = a^2 + b^2 + c^2 - 2ab + 2bc - 2ca$
- $(a + b)^3 = a^3 + 3a^2b + 3ab^2 + b^3$; $(a + b)^3 = a^3 + b^3 + 3ab(a + b)$
- $(a - b)^3 = a^3 - 3a^2b + 3ab^2 - b^3 = a^3 - b^3 - 3ab(a - b)$
- $a^3 - b^3 = (a - b)(a^2 + ab + b^2)$
- $a^3 + b^3 = (a + b)(a^2 - ab + b^2)$
- $(a + b)^4 = a^4 + 4a^3b + 6a^2b^2 + 4ab^3 + b^4$
- $(a - b)^4 = a^4 - 4a^3b + 6a^2b^2 - 4ab^3 + b^4$

PERCENTAGE

A percentage is a number or ratio which is expressed as a fraction of 100 and it is denoted by using '%' symbol.

$$\text{Percentage} = \frac{\text{Value obtained}}{\text{Total value}} \times 100$$

Example:

1. **A class of 120 students have 40 girls, rest of the students are boys. What is the percentage of boys in that class?**

Solution:

$$\text{Percentage} = \frac{\text{Value obtained}}{\text{Total value}} \times 100$$

$$\text{Total students} = \text{Total value} = 120$$

Total number of boys, for which percentage has to be calculated:

$$120–40 = 80$$

$$\text{Percentage of boys} = \frac{80}{10} \times 100 = 66.66\%$$

AVERAGE

The average or arithmetic mean is defined as the mean value which is equal to the ratio of the sum of a number of a given set of values to the total number of values present in the set.

$$\text{Average} = \frac{\text{Sum of observations}}{\text{Total number of observations}}$$

Some Important Point to Remember

- Average of the first 10 whole numbers is 4.5
- Average of the first 10 natural numbers is 5.5
- Average of the first 10 even numbers is 11
- Average of the first 10 odd numbers is 10

Example:

1. **Find the average of 2, 4, 6, 8, 10.**

Solution:

$$\text{Average} = \frac{\text{Sum of observations}}{\text{Total number of observations}}$$

$$\text{Sum of observations} = 2 + 4 + 6 + 8 + 10 = 30$$

$$\text{No. of Observations} = 5$$

By putting the values,

$$\text{Average} = \frac{30}{5}$$

$$\text{Average} = 6$$

PROFIT AND LOSS

Cost Price (CP): The price at which a product is purchased is called cost price.

Selling Price (SP): The price at which a product is sold is called the selling price.

Profit/Gain (P): If a product is sold at a price that is more than its cost price then the seller makes a profit.

Loss (L): If a product is sold at a price that is less than its cost price then the seller makes a loss.

Some Important Formula

- Profit, P = SP – CP; SP > CP
- Loss, L = CP – SP; CP > SP
- $P\% = (P/CP) \times 100$
- $L\% = (L/CP) \times 100$
- $SP = \{(100 + P\%)/100\} \times CP$
- $SP = \{(100 - L\%)/100\} \times CP$
- $CP = \{100/(100 + P\%)\} \times SP$
- $CP = \{100/(100 - L\%)\} \times SP$

Example:

1. **A man buys a shirt of ₹1000 and sells it at a loss of 15%. What is the selling price of the shirt?**

Solution:

Cost Price of the shirt is ₹1000

The loss percentage is 15%

As we know, Loss percentage = (Loss/Cost Price) × 100

15 = (Loss/1000) × 100

Therefore, Loss = 150 ₹

As we know,

Loss = Cost Price – Selling Price

So, Selling Price = Cost Price – Loss

= 1000 – 150

Selling Price = ₹850/-

So, selling price of the shirt is ₹850/-

2. **A man gains 30% by selling a watch for a certain price. If he sells it at double the current selling price, then what will be the profit percentage?**

Solution:

Let, the cost price be ₹ x.

∴ Selling price = ₹ 1.3x

Now, new SP = ₹ 2.6x

∴ Profit % = [(2.6x – x)] × 100 = 160%

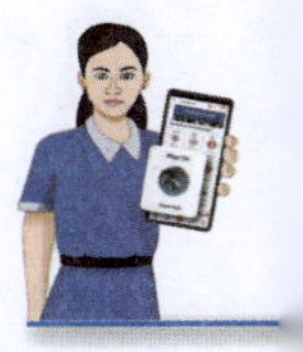

SIMPLE AND COMPOUND INTEREST

Simple Interest

Principal: It is a sum of money lent or invested, on which interest is paid after a certain period.
Interest: Interest is extra money paid on the principal.
Simple interest: It is a method to calculate the amount of interest charged on a sum at a given rate and given time period

Important Formula for Simple Interest

Simple Interest (SI) = (P × R × T)/100
Where, P = Principal,
R = Rate of Interest,
T = Time (Period).
The time is in years and the rate of interest is in percentage (%).

Compound Interest

Compound interest includes the principal and the interest gained on the previous year's principal.

When the compound interest is calculated annually:

$$\text{Amount} = P\left[1+\frac{R}{100}\right]^n$$

When the compound interest is calculated half-yearly:

$$\text{Amount} = P\left[1+\frac{R/2}{100}\right]^{2n}$$

When the compound interest is calculated Quarterly yearly:

$$\text{Amount} = P\left[1+\frac{R/4}{100}\right]^{4n}$$

When rates are different for different years, i.e., $R_{1\%}$, $R_{2\%}$, $R_{3\%}$ for 1st, 2nd and 3rd year respectively:

$$\text{Amount} = \left[1+\frac{R_1}{100}\right]\left[1+\frac{R_2}{100}\right]\left[1+\frac{R_3}{100}\right]$$

Example:

1. **At what rate of simple interest a certain sum of money doubled in 10 years?**

Solution:

Amount = Principal + Simple interest
Because the principal get doubled, so,
Amount = 2× Principal
2 × Principal = Principal + Simple interest
2P = P+SI
So, SI = P

$$P = \frac{P \times R \times 10}{100} = R = \frac{100}{10} = 10$$

2. **Find the compound interest (CI) on Rs. 12,000 for 2 years at 5% per annum compounded annually.**

Solution:

Given,
Principal (P) = Rs. 12,000
Rate (R) = 5
Number of years (n) = 2 years

$$\text{Amount} = P\left[1+\frac{R}{100}\right]^n$$

= 12000 [1 + (5/100)]²
= 12000 [1 + (1/20)]²
= 12000 [(20 + 1)/20]²
= 12000 × (21/20) × (21/20)
= 126 × 121 = 13230
Total amount, A = ₹13230
Compound interest (CI) = A – P
= ₹13230 – ₹12,000
= ₹1230

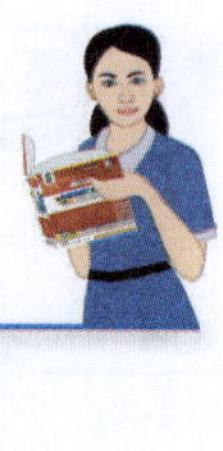

TIME AND WORK

Important Formula

- Work Done = Time Taken × Rate of Work
- Rate of Work = 1/Time Taken
- Time Taken = 1/Rate of Work
- If a piece of work is done in x number of days, then the work done in one day = 1/x
- Total Wok Done = Number of Days × Efficiency
- Efficiency and Time are inversely proportional to each other
- X:Y is the ratio of the number of men which are required to complete a piece of work, then the ratio of the time taken by them to complete the work will be y:x
- If x number of people can do W1 work, in D1 days, working T1 hours each day and the number of people can do W2 work, in D2 days, working T2 hours each day, then the relation between them will be

$$\frac{M1 \times D1 \times T1}{W1} = \frac{M2 \times D2 \times T2}{W2}$$

Example:

1. **Supriya can do a piece of work in 5 days and Khyati can do it in 6 days. How long will they take if they work together?**

Solution:

Supriya takes 5 days (x) and Khyati can takes 6 days (y)
If they work together, the time required to complete the work is
Supriya + Khyati = 1/x + 1/y = xy/(x+y)
= (5 × 6)/(5+6) = 30/11
= 2.73 days
So, If they work together they will do the work in 2.73 days

2. **Sugandha alone can do a job in 30 days. In how many days can Ruby alone do the job, if together they can do the job in 6 days?**

Solution:

⇒ Efficiency of **Sugandha** + **Ruby**
= (1/40) : (1/8) = 1 : 5
⇒ Efficiency of **Ruby**/Efficiency of **Sugandha**
= (5 – 1)/1 = 4/1
Ruby is 4 times efficient than **Sugandha**
⇒ Number of days taken by **Ruby** = 1/4 × Number of days taken by **Sugandha** = 40/4 = 10 days

TIME AND DISTANCE

Important Formula

- **Speed = Distance/Time**
- **Distance = Speed x Time** and
- **Time = Distance / Speed**
- **Conversion of km/hr into m/s**
  1 km/hr = 5/18 m/s
- **Conversion of m/s into km/hr**
  1 m/s = 18/5 km/hr
- **Average Velocity:** Suppose a boy covers a certain distance at v_1 km/h. and an equal distance at v_2 km/h. Then the average speed

during the whole journey is $\left(\frac{2v1v2}{v1+v2}\right)$

Suppose two girls are moving in the same direction at u m/s and v m/s respectively, then their relative speed = (u – v) m/s

Suppose two girls are moving in the opposite direction at u m/s and v m/s respectively, then their relative speed = (u + v) m/s

Example:

1. **If Shivani runs at a speed of 20 Km/hr, how much time does she take to cover a distance of 400 meters?**

Solution:

Aditya's speed = 20 km/hr = [20 × (5/18)]m/sec
= 50/9 m/sec

Time taken to cover 400 m = 400 ÷ 50/9
= 400 × 9/50 = 72 sec = 1.2 min

2. **Supriya travels from Noida to Delhi at the speed of 40 km/hr and she returns at the speed of 50 km/hr, what is the average speed of the journey?**

Solution:

Using the formula, $\left(\frac{2v1v2}{v1+v2}\right)$

$= \frac{2\times 40\times 50}{40+50} = \frac{4000}{90}$

= 44.44 km/hr

PIPES AND CISTERNS

Important Formula

- If it takes x hours to fill up a tank, then tank filled in 1 hr = 1/x
- If it takes y hours to empty the tank, then tank emptied in 1 hour
- = 1/y
- If a pipe fills a tank in x hours and empties the same tank in y hours if both the pipes are opened at the same time, then the net part of the tank filled in 1 hr = {(xy)/(y–x)}, provided y > x
- If a pipe fills a tank in x hours and empties the same tank in y hours if both the pipes are opened at the same time, then the net part of the tank filled in 1 hr = {(xy)/(x–y)}, provided x>y
- Net work done = (Sum of work done by Inlets) – (Sum of work done by Outlets)
- One inlet fills the tank in x hours and the other inlet fills the same tank in y hours, if both the inlets are opened at the same time, the time taken to fill the whole tank = {(xy)/(y + x)}
- If two pipes take x and y hours respectively to fill a tank of water and a third pipe is opened which takes z hours to empty the tank, then the time taken to fill the tank = {1/(1/x) + (1/y) + (1/z)} and the net part of the tank filled in 1 hr = (1/x) + (1/y) – (1/z)

Example:

1. **If three pipes, P, Q and R take 14 hours to fill a tank. After working together for 2 hours, R was closed and, P and Q filled the remaining tank in 7 hours. How many hours would it take R alone to fill the tank?**

Solution:

Part of the tank which was filled in 2 hours = 2/6 = ⅓

The part of the tank remaining to be filled = 1 – ⅓ = ⅔

Work done by P and Q together in 7 hours = ⅔

Work done by P and Q together in 1 hour = [(⅔)/7] = 2/21

Work done by R in 1 hour
= [{(X+Y + X)'s 1 hour's work} – {(X + Y)'s 1 hour's work}]
= (⅙) – (2/21) = 1/14

Therefore, R alone will fill the tank in 14 hours.

BOATS AND STEAMS

Some Concepts related to Boats and Streams

- **Stream:** Running river water is known as stream.
- **Upstream:** If the boat moves in the opposite direction of the flow of the stream then it is said that the boat is moving upstream. In this case, the boat's net speed is upstream speed.
- **Downstream:** If the boat moves along the direction of the flow of the stream then it is said that the boat is moving downstream. In this case, the boat's net speed is downstream speed.
- **Still Water:** Stationary water is known as still water. It happens when the speed of the water is zero.

Some Important Formula

- **Upstream = (u–v) km/hr,** where "u" is the speed of the boat in still water and "v" is the speed of the stream
- **Downstream = (u+v) km/hr,** where "u" is the speed of the boat in still water and "v" is the speed of the stream
- **Speed of Boat in Still Water = ½ (Downstream Speed + Upstream Speed)**
- **Speed of Stream = ½ (Downstream Speed – Upstream Speed)**

Example:

1. **Speed of a speedboat is 15 km/hr in still water goes 30 km downstream and it comes back in 4 hours 30 minutes. What is the speed of the stream in km/hr?**

Solution:

Let the speed of the stream be x km/hr

Upstream Speed = 15 + x

Downstream Speed = 15 – x

So, {30/(15 + x)} + {30/(15 – x)} = 4½ (4 hours 30 minutes)

⇒ {900/(225 – x^2)} = 9/2

⇒ $9x^2 = 225$

⇒ $x^2 = 25$

⇒ x = 5

PROBLEMS BASED ON TRAIN

Some Important Formula

- If two trains 'P' and 'Q' have lengths 'x' and 'y' and their speeds are 'a' and 'b', respectively, and moving in the same direction. Then:

  Time taken by both the trains to cross each other = (a + b)/(x – y) and their **relative speed** = x – y.

  For trains moving in the opposite direction, Time taken by both the trains to cross each other = (a + b)/(x + y) and **relative speed** = x + y.
- If the train of length 'x' with speed 'a' is moving and passes a stationary object, then the time taken by the train to cross the object = x/a.
- If the train of length 'x' with speed 'a' is moving and passes the bridge/platform of length 'y', then the time taken by the train to cross the bridge/platform = ((x + y)/a).

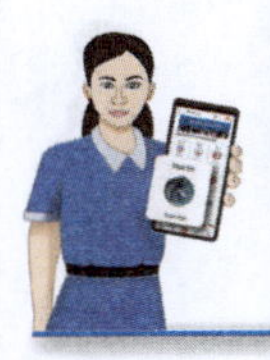

Example:

1. **A train 'A' which is moving at a speed of 90 km/hr and crosses another train 'B' which is moving in the same direction at 180 km/hr in 30 seconds. What is the sum of the lengths of the two trains?**

Solution:

Speed of train B = 180 km/hr = [180 × (5/18)] = 50 m/sec.
Trains are moving in the same direction.
Hence,
Relative speed = (50 – 25) m/sec = 25 m/sec
Time taken by train A to cross train B = 30 sec
The sum of the length of the trains = distance traveled
Distance = Speed × Time = (25 × 30) = 750 m
Hence, the Sum of the length of the train = 750 m.

MENSURATION

Mensuration is the branch of mathematics that deals with the measurement of length, area, volume, surface area, lateral surface area of different geometrical shapes.

AREA/PERIMETER

Important Formulae

1. a. Area of a rectangle = length × breadth
   b. Perimeter = 2(length + breadth)
2. Area of a square = Side × Side = $\frac{1}{2}$(diagonal)^2
3. Area of 4 walls of a room = 2 (length + breadth) × height
4. Area of a triangle = $\frac{1}{2}$ × base × height
5. Area of a triangle = $\sqrt{s(s-a)(s-b)(s-c)}$
   Where a, b, c are the sides of triangle.
6. Area of an equilateral triangle = $\frac{\sqrt{3}}{4}$ × (side)^2
7. Area of a triangle = $\frac{1}{2}$ ab sin Θ
   Where 'a' and 'b' are the lengths of triangle and Θ is the angle between them.
8. Area of a parallelogram = base × height
9. Area of a rhombus = $\frac{1}{2}$ × (Products of diagonals)
10. Area of a trapezium = $\frac{1}{2}$ × (Products of parallel sides) × height
11. Area of a circle = πr^2
12. Circumference of a circle = $2\pi r$

Example:

1. **The area of a trapezium is 540 m², the distance between the parallel sides is 12 m and one of the parallel sides is 30 m. Find the other parallel side.**

Solution:

One of the parallel sides of the trapezium is a = 30 m, let another parallel side be b, height h = 12 m.
The given area of trapezium = 540 m^2
We know, by formula;
Area of a trapezium = ½ h (a + b)
540 = ½(12) (30 + b)
30 + b = (540 × 2)/12
b = 90 – 30 = 60 m

2. **A cylinder whose radius is 7 cm and total surface area is 968 cm², what will be its height?**

Solution:

Let height of the cylinder = h, radius = r = 7 cm
Total surface area = 2πr (h + r)
TSA = 2 × (22/7) × 7 × (7 + h) = 968 h = 15 cm

3. **A rhombus whose diagonals are of length 24 cm and 40 cm, respectively, what will be its area?**

Solution:

d_1 = 24 cm
d_2 = 40 cm
Area of rhombus = ½ d_1 d_2
A = ½ × 24 × 40
A = 480 cm^2

VOLUME AND SURFACE AREA

Important Formulae

Name of the solid	Curved surface area	Total surface area	Volume
Cuboid	2h(l + b)	2(lb + bh + hl)	lbh
Cube	4a^2	6a^2	a^3
Right circular cylinder	$2\pi rh$	$2\pi r(r + h)$	$\pi r^2 h$
Right circular cone	πrl	$2\pi r(r + l)$	$\frac{1}{3}\pi r^2 h$
Sphere	–	$4\pi r^2$	$\frac{4}{3}\pi r^2$
Hemisphere	$2\pi r^2$	3pr2	$\frac{2}{3}\pi r^2$
Frustum of a cone	$\pi(r_1 + r_2)/l$ where l = $\sqrt{h^2 + (r_1 - r_2)^2}$	$\pi(r_1 + r_2)l + \pi r_1^2 + \pi r_2^2$	$\frac{1}{3}\pi h(\pi r_1^2 + \pi r_2^2 + r_1 r_2)$

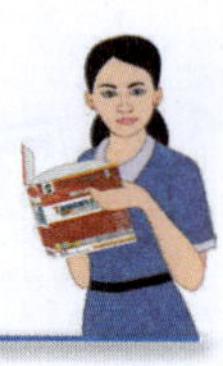

Example:

1. Find the total surface area of a cylinder with radius of base 3.5 cm and the height 20 cm.

Solution:

Radius = 3.5 cm

Height = 20 cm

Total surface area = $2\pi rh + 2\pi r^2 = 2\pi r(h + r)$

$$= \left[2 \times \frac{22}{7} \times 3.5 \times (20 + 3.5)\right]$$

= 517 cm^2

2. A hemisphere whose surface area is 50 sq. inches. Find its volume.

Solution:

The surface area of hemisphere = 50 sq. inches

The formula of Surface area of the hemisphere = $2\pi r^2$

$50 = 2\pi r^2$

$r^2 = 50/2\pi$ ($\pi = 3.14$) = 7.96

r = 2.82

The radius of the hemisphere is 2.82 inches

Volume of a hemisphere = $2\ \pi r^3/3$ cubic units

$= 2/3 \times 3.14 \times (2.82)^3$

$= 2/3 \times 3.14 \times 22.43$

$= 2/3 \times 70.43 = 46.96$

The volume of the hemisphere is 46.96 cm^3

3. If radius and height of a cone are 4 cm and 3 cm respectively then find its area.

Solution:

Given, radius of cone = 4 cm and height of cone = 3 cm.

As per the formula of area of cone, we know;

Slant height = $l = \sqrt{(4^2 + 3^2)} = \sqrt{25} = 5$ cm

Area = $\pi r(r + l)$

= (22/7) × 4(4 + 5)

= (22/7)36

= 113. 14 cm^2

PRACTICE QUESTIONS

1. **If the product of three consecutive integers is 120, then the sum of the integers is:**
   a. 9 b. 12
   c. 14 d. 15
2. **A man can row $\frac{3}{4}$ of a km against the stream in $11\frac{1}{4}$ minutes and return in $7\frac{1}{2}$ minutes, find the speed of the man in still water.**
   a. 3 km/hr b. 4 km/hr
   c. 5 km/hr d. 6 km/hr
3. **The profit earned by selling an article for 832 is equal to the loss incurred when the same article is sold for 448. What should be the sale price for making 50% profit?**
   a. 920 b. 960
   c. 1060 d. 1200
4. **The ratio between the length and the breadth of a rectangular park is 3:2. If a man cycling along the boundary of the park at the speed of 12 km/hr completes one round in 8 minutes, then the area of the park (in sq. m) is:**
   a. 15360 sq. m b. 153600 sq. m
   c. 30720 sq. m d. 307200 sq. m
5. **If the selling price is doubled, the profit triples. Find the profit percent.**
   a. 150% b. 200%
   c. 100% d. 400%
6. **A father is now three times as old as his son. Five years back, he was four times as old as his son. What is the age of the son is:**
   a. 12 b. 15
   c. 18 d. 20
7. **If 35% of a number is 175, then what percent of 175 is that number?**
   a. 35%
   b. 65%
   c. 280%
   d. None of the above
8. **An airplane covers a certain distance at a speed of 240 km/h in 5 hours. To cover the same distance in $1\frac{2}{3}$ hours, it must travel at a speed of:**
   a. 300 km/h b. 360 km/h
   c. 600 km/h d. 720 km/h
9. **The perimeter of a rectangular field is 480 meters and the ratio between the length and the breadth is 5:3 the area is:**
   a. 1350 sq. m b. 1550 sq. m
   c. 13500 sq. m d. 15500 sq. m
10. **A star is 8.1 × 10^{13} km away from the earth. Suppose light travels at the speed of 3.0 × 10^5 km per second how long will it take the light from the star to reach the earth?**
    a. 7.5 ×10^3 hours b. 7.5 × 10^4 hours
    c. 2.7 × 10^{10} seconds d. 2.7 × 10^{11} seconds
11. **Today is Amit's birthday. One year from today he will be twice as old as he was 12 years ago. Find the current age of Amit.**
    a. 18 years b. 16 years
    c. 22 years d. 25 years
12. **If a: b: c = 2 : 4 : 6, then the ratio of (a + b + c) : c is equal to:**
    a. 2:1 b. 1:2
    c. 3:2 d. 2:3
13. **The C.P. of an article is 20% of the S.P. The percent that the S.P. is of C.P. is**
    a. 250 b. 240
    c. 500 d. 40
14. **8 out of 2400 parts of a container is water. What is the fraction of water in the container?**
    a. $\frac{1}{3}$ b. $\frac{11}{50}$
    c. $\frac{1}{45}$ d. $\frac{2}{45}$
15. **The simple interest at 5% for 2 years will be ₹200 on a sum of:**
    a. ₹500 b. ₹20000
    c. ₹2000 d. ₹1000
16. **Find the average of the following sets of scores: 567, 234, 467, 123, 324, 345, 601**
    a. 380 b. 426
    c. 652 d. 257

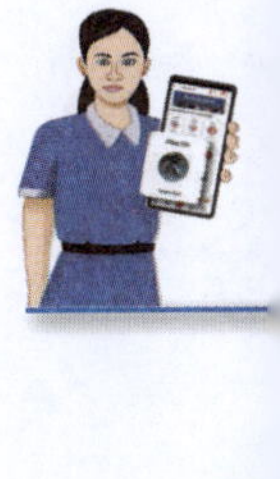

17. The length of a room is 6 m and the width is 4 m. Find the cost of paving the floor by slab at the rate of ₹600 per square meter.

a. 15670
b. 14400
c. 15390
d. 14290

18. 15% of 578 + 22.5 % of 644 is:

a. 241.7
b. 238.98
c. 231.60
d. 237.65

Practice Exercises

Answers

1.	d	2.	c	3.	b	4.	b	5.	c	6.	b	7.	d	8.	d	9.	c	10.	b
11.	c	12.	a	13.	c	14.	a	15.	c	16.	a	17.	b	18.	c				

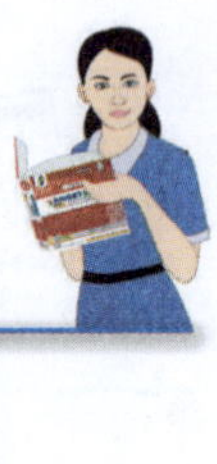